100 Questions & Answers About Liver Cancer

Ghassan K. Abou-Alfa, MD
Memorial Sloan-Kettering Cancer Center

Ronald DeMatteo, MD
Memorial Sloan-Kettering Cancer Center

JONES AND BARTLETT PUBLISHERS
Sudbury, Massachusetts
BOSTON   TORONTO   LONDON   SINGAPORE

BC Cancer Agency
CARE & RESEARCH

While the BC Cancer Agency considers this information
to be useful, it may vary from our standard practice and
protocol.

It is intended for educational purposes only and should
not be substituted for the advice of a healthcare
professional.

World Headquarters

Jones and Bartlett
Publishers
40 Tall Pine Drive
Sudbury, MA 01776
info@jbpub.com
www.jbpub.com

Jones and Bartlett
Publishers Canada
6339 Ormindale Way
Mississauga, ON L5V 1J2
CANADA

Jones and Bartlett
Publishers International
Barb House, Barb Mews
London W6 7PA
UK

Jones and Bartlett's books and products are available through most bookstores and online book-sellers. To contact Jones and Bartlett Publishers directly, call 800-832-0034, fax 978-443-8000, or visit our website www.jbpub.com.

Substantial discounts on bulk quantities of Jones and Bartlett's publications are available to corporations, professional associations, and other qualified organizations. For details and specific discount information, contact the special sales department at Jones and Bartlett via the above contact information or send an email to specialsales@jbpub.com.

Library of Congress Cataloging-in-Publication Data
Abou-Alfa, Ghassan K.
  100 questions and answers about liver cancer / Ghassan K. Abou-Alfa
and Ronald DeMatteo.
    p. cm.
  Includes bibliographical references and index.
  ISBN 0-7637-4754-8 (pbk.)
  1. Liver—Cancer—Popular works. I. DeMatteo, Ronald. II. Title.
  III. Title: One hundred questions and answers about liver cancer.
  RC280.L5A26 2006
  616.99'436—dc22
                          2005012145

The authors, editor, and publisher have made every effort to provide accurate information. However, they are not responsible for errors, omissions, or for any outcomes related to the use of the contents of this book and take no responsibility for the use of the products described. Treatments and side effects described in this book may not be applicable to all patients; likewise, some patients may require a dose or experience a side effect that is not described herein. The reader should confer with his or her own physician regarding specific treatments and side effects. Drugs and medical devices are discussed that may have limited availability controlled by the Food and Drug Administration (FDA) for use only in a research study or clinical trial. The drug information presented has been derived from reference sources, recently published data, and pharmaceutical research data. Research, clinical practice, and government regulations often change the accepted standard in this field. When consideration is being given to use of any drug in the clinical setting, the health care provider or reader is responsible for determining FDA status of the drug, reading the package insert, reviewing prescribing information for the most up-to-date recommendations on dose, precautions, and contraindications, and determining the appropriate usage for the product. This is especially important in the case of drugs that are new or seldom used.

Production Credits
Executive Publisher: Chris Davis
Production Director: Amy Rose
Production Assistant: Alison Meier
Editorial Assistant: Kathy Richardson
Marketing Associate: Laura Kavigian
Manufacturing Buyer: Therese Connell
Cover Design: Rebecca Senecal
Composition: Northeast Compositors
Printing and Binding: Malloy Inc.
Cover Printing: Malloy Inc.

Printed in the United States of America
09 08 07 06 05   10 9 8 7 6 5 4 3 2 1

To Our Patients and Their Families

Contents

Primary liver cancer is a very common form of cancer worldwide often associated with existing liver failure or cirrhosis. Before you were diagnosed with cancer, you might have been told a few years earlier that you have liver cirrhosis from hepatitis, alcohol use, or some other reason, and thus you may be at risk for developing primary liver cancer.

Dealing with liver cancer is a very complex matter, especially when it comes to medical care, as many specialists may be involved. You can expect to be treated by a gastroenterologist, a hepatologist regarding the liver cirrhosis, and many other specialists treating the cancer itself. These may include a surgeon, a medical oncologist, a transplant surgeon, an interventional radiologist, and a radiation therapist, among others.

One of the reasons we decided to write this book was to help you understand and coordinate your care among all those specialists. We also felt an important need for patients with liver cancer to understand all the available therapies, especially as new ones emerge frequently.

This book will also be of help in better understanding this cancer and all the signs and symptoms that may occur. We emphasize the management of symptoms like pain or leg swelling in an attempt to ensure comfort to all patients who are battling the disease. It is also an excellent resource for social issues that may arise as a result of the cancer. You will find information on how to handle fear, family concerns, work issues, and many other topics. Resources of all kinds, including web sites, are listed.

We hope that you, your family, and friends find the answers and comfort you need through reading this book. Knowledge empowers, and as more advocates sound their voice, we believe this will help raise awareness in the battle against liver cancer.

The Authors

Acknowledgment

The authors and publisher gratefully acknowledge the contribution provided by Mr. Paul Borkowski, whose comments appear in the front of the book.

We would also like to extend our sincere appreciation to Mr. Sam Hou for graciously contributing his comments. Together with his family, Sam helped with the care of his father, Derson Hou, who was diagnosed with primary liver cancer in December 1999. While undergoing embolization and alcohol injection treatments at Memorial Sloan-Kettering Cancer Center, Derson experienced the daily joy of playing with his two new grandsons, Ryan and Samuel. He passed away peacefully in February 2004.

Around Thanksgiving of 2003, my yearly battle with bronchitis and the usual upper respiratory complications began. I visited my primary care physician and started on a regimen of antibiotics. I had a history of emphysema and had contracted pneumonia on three separate occasions. In many ways, this felt familiar. Because I did not get any better in two weeks, we moved to the second step, an appointment with my pulmonologist. Something was different this time because the usual tests did not produce the usual answers. I still had trouble catching my breath and was very fatigued all of the time even though my cough was gone. My lung specialist sent me to get a lung CT scan. In the meantime, we made an appointment with my cardiologist to enlist his input about the problem. He must have seen something unusual in my symptoms because he recommended a whole-body CT scan with contrast. To be thorough, we made an appointment with my gastroenterologist.

The CT scan results were ready at the same time as my appointment with my gastroenterologist. He accessed the results while we were in his office. As it turned out, he was the one who told us the news. I can still remember sitting in his exam room when he came in with the results of my CT scan; I asked him to give us some good news. Instead, he said, "It seems that you have cancer." At that moment, the roof fell in on us. Then our journey with the "Big C" began.

Living on Long Island's South Shore, we proceeded to see an oncology group connected with South Side Hospital. The doctor was very nice and helpful. He had done his internship at Memorial Sloan-Kettering Cancer Center and concurred with our plan to go to that institution for evaluation. He read the CT scan report that stated that I probably had a type of liver cancer known as hepatocellular carcinoma. His approach essentially consisted of offering palliative care. This approach seemed to be too passive; everyone we talked to said that because we lived on Long Island we had the option of going to the close-by Memorial Sloan-Kettering Cancer Center in Manhattan. This turned out to be very true in our case.

Our journey began on January 2004 with our first visit to Memorial Sloan-Kettering Cancer Center. We had an appointment with a specialist to check the tumor near my lung. He assessed the tumors and said that it was basically a "slam dunk" to remove the tumor on my rib cage; however, he deferred to another specialist because the site of the liver tumor seemed to be primary. The liver surgeon told me that I was not a candidate for a transplant or surgery because my cancer had already moved to other organs, or metastasized. He added, "If you don't do anything, all you have is about a year to live." I did not appreciate hearing that as I had no intention of "doing nothing." We were then sent to Dr. Abou-Alfa to explore the available options. Since the first time we met Dr. Abou-Alfa, I liked him. He seemed to know his stuff! He was patient and kind, as well as very competent. His staff seemed very capable and dealt admirably with any and all questions that we had. It is very important to find the right doctor. Obviously, it is imperative to find someone who sees enough cases to develop skill and expertise. The type of cancer that I have is not too common in this country; consequently, the "neighborhood" doctors that I saw had an insufficient frame of reference for what my options actually were.

When you learn that you have cancer—no matter what type—your world seems to do a 180-degree turn. A lot of feelings seem to rise up—both good and bad! A lot of "wouldas, shouldas, and couldas" come up. As far as my life is concerned, the paths that some of these feelings and emotions took could have proven to be dangerous ground, leading to isolation, depression, or apathy. Luckily, I have the ability to surround myself with positive people and to keep my own outlook vital and upbeat. Many things in life just do not seem that important anymore or have to take a back seat to what is going on today.

At 57 years old, I found myself needing to take a long, hard look at my life. A lot of really tough decisions would have to be made that would affect not only my life but the lives of my family members as well. I had to re-evaluate much in my life if I was to have any chance against this disease. I certainly was not going to lie down and give in to it.

First, I had to re-evaluate my relationship with my God, whom I had taken for granted until this point. Also, my family and friends had to be seen in a different light. Since all of this came about, my family has really closed ranks around me, and I have found out who my real friends are. They are the ones who do not treat me as if I have the pox! I am *not* my cancer!

I have also come to believe in the "power of prayer." A great feeling of peace and serenity can come from prayer and meditation. Every day the prayer lines remain open. A lot of angels—both seen and unseen—in my life have helped me with my burdens. Whether or not I am willing or able to ask for help, it seems that help is there anyway. I am truly grateful for this. All of my angels know who they are.

I also found many things that I still needed to do in my life in order to stand a chance with my disease. I had to retire from my job of 32 years with the United States Postal Service. That was a huge change in my daily routine, but it freed my time for treatment. Clouds often have silver linings, and retiring was an example of that truth for me. Education and knowledge became priorities for me, and they should for you, too. I found that there was much more to cancer than I as a lay person knew. I needed to find out as much as I could about my type of cancer. Questions such as these arose: Am I eligible for a liver transplant? If not, why? Why was I so constantly fatigued? What effect did my blood counts have on treatment? Decisions had to be made about whether to take part in a clinical trial or to go with standard treatment. I got a crash course in the phases of a clinical trial and how to negotiate web sites to determine what trials were being offered. We spoke to researchers, doctors, and medical personnel around the country. After weighing all of the pros and cons, I decided to seek treatment at Memorial Sloan-Kettering Cancer Center. The Internet was a great help as an overall resource, although it was overwhelming at times. Dr. Abou-Alfa and his very knowledgeable staff were there to answer all my questions—and I had questions about everything! This book put together by Drs. Abou-Alfa and DeMatteo can be an invaluable tool in our search for answers to questions that we may have about my type of liver cancer (hepatocellular carcinoma). It does a great job of answering questions about why I got the type of liver cancer I have, how common it is, and where it comes from. This book covers other basics, such as how doctors test for hepatocellular carcinoma after the symptoms are detected. It discusses how to cope with the diagnosis and what treatment options are available. How important is it to discuss these options with your physician to determine which is best for you? This book takes a very concise and thorough look at all avenues that pertain to hepatocellular carcinoma, its causes and effects, its diagnosis and treatment, as well as all of the practical issues right down to end-of-life issues.

To end on a good note! I am still here. It has been over a year, and I plan to keep on battling! I have found that I do not have to be alone in this battle, and neither does anyone else. My heartfelt thanks go to Dr. Abou-Alfa and Dr. DeMatteo and their staff for all of their help and support. I am grateful to God for always being there. My deepest appreciation goes to my great wife and family and all of the angels in my life; their love and prayers are always accepted (humbly). To my fellow cancer patients, whose shared knowledge has made this journey possible and worthwhile: you have a special place in my heart. There is nothing like taking the journey with someone who knows what it feels like to walk in your shoes. I feel tremendous love and gratitude to each person in my circle of support. If I can help just one other person I have done my part. Please do not ever give up hope, even when things seem to be at their darkest. A good attitude and a good sense of humor are golden tools to have in our corner. Try not to forget who is really in charge. I know I had a tendency to forget. I believe that is part of being human. Remember that prayer has the ability to move mountains, and miracles do happen!

Paul J. Borkowski

PART ONE

The Basics

What is the liver?

What is liver cancer?

Are there different types of liver cancer?

More ...

Liver

an organ located in the upper right-hand side of the abdomen; responsible for making proteins and removing toxins and wastes from the body.

Proteins

essential body substances that include enzymes, hormones, antibodies, and other substances that are critical for the functioning of the human body.

Bile

a collection of salts and proteins that is made by the liver and carried by the bile duct to the gallbladder and the intestine. Bile is green and gives feces their brown color.

Intestine

the part of the gastrointestinal tract between the stomach and rectum. The intestine helps digest food and regulate water, certain vitamins, and salts of the body.

Cells

the smallest structural unit of a living organism that is capable of functioning independently.

1. What is the liver?

The **liver** is the largest organ in the body. It weighs approximately 1.5 kilograms (or over 3 pounds). It resides in the upper abdomen on the right-hand side. Because most of the liver is underneath and protected by the right rib cage, you normally cannot feel it. The liver has numerous functions (Table 1). It is responsible for making many different **proteins**. It can be thought of as the furnace of the body because it is the primary source of energy. It also acts as a filter to remove wastes and toxins from our blood. The liver makes **bile**, which empties into the **intestine**. Bile contains waste products as well as substances that help us to digest fat (Table 1).

2. What is liver cancer?

Like any other organ, the liver is made of a basic element called **cells**. Cells are the smallest structural unit of a living organism. Cells are born and die, and thus, the body is always in need of new cells to replenish the older and dead ones. This is a very tightly regulated phenomenon in the body. In certain instances, a cell becomes capable of dividing in an uncontrolled fashion, and a **cancer** may then form and grow. Although the cells of a certain organ such as the liver are highly specialized and perform the tasks that are assigned to them, a **tumor** can lose some of its normal functions and/or acquire other new functions. One of the functions that cancer cells can acquire is the ability to grow and invade into the healthy parts of the same organ or a neighboring one. Cancer cells can also steal the blood supply from normal tissue in order to grow larger. Cancer cells may even travel distances to other

Table 1   Functions of the Liver

Stores energy in the form of sugar and carbohydrates

Maintains normal blood sugar levels

Breaks down fat

Makes protein

Stores vitamins A, D, and B12

Makes proteins that help blood clot

Stores iron

Removes drugs and toxins from the blood

Produces cholesterol

Makes bile

Helps to protect your body from infection

The Basics

organs or places in the body to establish new tumors. This process is called **metastasis**.

3. Are there different types of liver cancer?

Two broad categories of liver cancer exist: primary and secondary (Table 2). **Primary liver cancer** means that the tumor originated in the liver. A tumor can start from any of the different types of cells that normally exist in the liver. **Hepatocellular cancer** is the most common type of primary liver cancer. It is also known as **hepatocellular carcinoma** or **hepatoma** for short and is often abbreviated HCC. Hepatocellular cancer arises from **hepatocytes**, which are the cells that are responsible for most of the functions listed in Table 1.

There is a subtype of hepatocellular cancer called **fibrolamellar hepatocellular carcinoma**. It makes up less than 5% of all hepatocellular cancers. It tends to occur in young adults and is typically not associated

Cancer

the uncontrolled replication of cells that leads to abnormal growth that may invade local organs or tissues or may travel to other places in the body.

Tumor

a cancerous growth.

Metastasis

the spread of cancer beyond its primary location.

Primary liver cancer

cancer that originates within the liver.

Hepatocellular cancer

a type of primary liver cancer that originates in hepatocytes, a type of liver cell.

3

Table 2 Types of Liver Cancer

Primary liver cancer	Hepatocellular cancer
	Cholangiocarcinoma
	Mixed hepatocellular and cholangio-carcinoma
	Hepatoblastoma
	Gallbladder cancer
Secondary liver cancer	From colon, breast, pancreas, or other cancers

Hepatocellular carcinoma
cancer of the liver cells, a type of primary liver cancer.

Hepatoma
short name for hepatocellular carcinoma.

Hepatocytes
liver cells.

Fibrolamellar hepatocellular carcinoma
a variant of hepatoma that occurs typically in young adults.

Cholangio-carcinoma
cancer of the bile ducts.

Hepatoblastoma
a rare type of primary liver cancer that occurs in children.

Gallbladder
a storage tank for bile.

with an underlying liver disease. In general, it carries a better prognosis.

The other types of primary liver cancer are rare. **Cholangiocarcinoma** is a cancer that arises from the bile ducts within the liver. Mixed hepatocellular and cholangiocarcinoma is a tumor that contains elements of both hepatocellular cancer and cholangiocarcinoma. **Hepatoblastoma** is a primary liver cancer that occurs in children. Cancer can also arise in the **gallbladder**. A variety of other very rare primary liver tumors exist.

Secondary liver cancer means that the cancer started somewhere else in the body. Many cancers, like those of the colon, breast, and pancreas, can spread, or metastasize, to the liver. These patients do not have "liver cancer" in the way that doctors use the phrase. Instead, they have metastases to their liver. For example, if a breast cancer spreads to the liver, it is called metastatic breast cancer and is not referred to as liver cancer.

4. Which type of liver cancer is this book about?

In this book, we answer questions about only hepatocellular cancer, the most common type of primary liver cancer. This book is not written to answer questions about other types of primary liver cancer or secondary liver cancers.

Secondary liver cancer

cancers that started in other organs of the body and have traveled to the liver.

The Basics

PART TWO

Risk Factors

Is hepatocellular cancer common?

Who is at risk for developing liver cancer?

What is liver cirrhosis?

More . . .

5. Is hepatocellular cancer common?

About 15,000 new cases of hepatocellular cancer are seen in the United States per year. It is uncommon compared with many other tumors. However, the frequency of the disease has increased by 75% in this country over the last decade, especially because of increased incidence of **hepatitis** C (see Question 9). In contrast, hepatocellular cancer is one of the most common tumors in the world, with nearly a million new people affected per year. This is largely because of its association with **chronic viral hepatitis**, explained in question 8.

6. Who is at risk for developing liver cancer?

Liver cancer can occur spontaneously for no apparent reason or can start because of an existing abnormality in the liver. Five main reasons exist for having an abnormal liver: (1) **viral hepatitis**, (2) alcohol use, (3) inherited **metabolic diseases** that affect the liver, (4) environmental factors, and (5) obesity and **diabetes**. Severe damage to the liver from the first four of these risk factors may result in **cirrhosis**.

7. What is liver cirrhosis?

Liver cirrhosis is basically the replacement of many normal liver cells with scar tissue and a loss of the normal arrangement of the remaining liver cells. It generally takes years of liver damage for cirrhosis to occur. Cirrhosis always affects the entire liver—not just one part

Hepatitis

inflammation of the liver. It may be caused by a variety of agents, including viruses, excessive alcohol use, metabolic diseases, and environmental toxins.

Chronic viral hepatitis

continuous state of infection during which the liver continues to be inflamed and may ultimately cause cirrhosis and cancer.

Viral hepatitis

inflammatory condition of the liver caused by an infection with a hepatitis virus.

Metabolic diseases

diseases in which the metabolism of a certain product may be impaired. They are usually genetically inherited.

Diabetes

a disease condition in which the body is unable to control sugar levels. In some instances, diabetes may lead to multiple complications and other diseases, and possibly is primary liver cancer.

of it. Cirrhosis is irreversible. A liver **transplantation** is the only way of getting rid of cirrhosis. Patients with cirrhosis are at particular risk for developing hepatocellular cancer. Although cirrhosis is a common precursor to liver cancer, many patients develop hepatocellular cancer without ever having cirrhosis (see Figure 1).

8. What is viral hepatitis?

The first risk factor for liver cancer that we consider is viral hepatitis. Hepatitis just means inflammation of the liver. Different types of viruses that infect humans and damage the liver cause viral hepatitis. Viruses infect humans in order to divide and grow because they cannot do so on their own. The most common hepatitis viruses are named A, B, and C. Hepatitis A is caused by the hepatitis A virus. Hepatitis B and C are caused by the hepatitis B and hepatitis C viruses.

Acute viral hepatitis means that a patient has recently become infected with the hepatitis A, B, or C virus. The patient may have a number of symptoms, including **fatigue**, loss of appetite, abdominal discomfort, **jaundice** (yellow color of the eyes or skin), and other abnormal liver blood tests. The treatment of acute viral

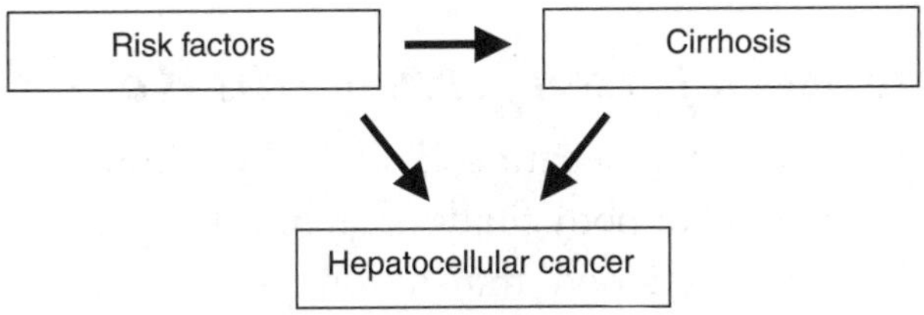

Risk Factors

Cirrhosis
condition in which normal liver tissue is replaced with scarred tissue. It is often associated with varied levels of loss of liver functions.

Transplantation
the removal of a patient's entire liver and replacement with part or all of the liver from another person. The other person may be alive (live donor) or just deceased (cadaveric donor).

Acute viral hepatitis
an active infection caused by a hepatitis virus.

Figure 1 Relationship of risk factors for hepatocellular cancer to cirrhosis and cancer development.

Fatigue

physical tiredness.

Jaundice

yellowish discoloration of the skin and eyes caused by accumulation of bilirubin.

hepatitis is just supportive care of the patient. Most patients fully recover, and most even completely forget about the illness.

After infection with the hepatitis A virus, the patient completely clears the virus from his or her body and is not at increased risk for cirrhosis or liver cancer. In contrast, some of the patients infected with the hepatitis B or C virus become chronically infected. In other words, they never completely remove the virus from their bodies. Patients with chronic hepatitis B or C are at risk for developing cirrhosis and all of its potential complications (see Question 22), including hepatocellular cancer.

The chance of developing chronic hepatitis B depends on the age of the patient at the time of acute viral infection. Chronic disease will develop in approximately 90% of newborns, 25% of children, and 10% of adults. There are 1.2 million people with chronic hepatitis B in the United States and 350 million worldwide. The frequency of chronic hepatitis B is expected to decrease now that there is an effective vaccine against it. Hepatitis C infection leads to chronic hepatitis in 55% to 85% of patients that are infected; 2.7 million patients have chronic hepatitis C in the United States.

Screening

studies and evaluations that attempt to identify a predisease state or an early form of disease, aiming at controlling it before it becomes advanced.

9. How does a person get hepatitis B or C?

People may contract hepatitis B or C by coming in contact with blood or body fluids of an infected patient. People who had a blood transfusion prior to 1992, before routine **screening** of blood products for hepatitis C was performed, may have gotten hepatitis C. Nowadays, it is extremely rare to get either form of chronic hepatitis from a blood transfusion. Contact with contaminated needles by intravenous drug users, health care workers, or people getting tattoos, is another mode of transmission. Two other routes of exposure, especially in the case of hepatitis B, are when unprotected sexual contact occurs with infected patients or when an infected mother transmits hepatitis to her newborn child during birth. Perinatal exposure is most common in East Asia, whereas blood and sexual exposure are more common methods of transmission in Europe and North America. The highest incidence of hepatitis B is in Sub-Saharan Africa, where close encounter among toddlers contributes to its high frequency in this area of the world. In the United States, hepatitis C viral infection is a major contributor to the risk of developing liver cancer. In Africa and Asia, hepatitis B infection is the predominant virus that contributes to the development of liver cancer.

My father was diagnosed with chronic hepatitis B about 3 to 4 years before his liver cancer was detected in 2000. His primary doctor had run a routine blood checkup and notified him that the hepatitis B screen came back positive. All of the immediate family members were then tested for the virus. My mother had already developed protective antibodies, whereas my siblings and I tested negative for the virus. As a precaution, we then all received the newly developed vaccines for both hepatitis A and B.

Although we can never be 100% certain, my father most likely contracted the virus during a blood transfusion during childhood in China and Taiwan before immigrating to

d States in 1966. Hepatitis and liver cancer are still
e prevalent in Asian countries than in the West.

me of his hepatitis diagnosis, we were told there
ing that could cure the hepatitis or reverse his
hosis. Later, we did come across one possible treat-
Hepatitis B: Epivir® (lamivudine). In retrospect,
I do not think that we realized that he was at much higher
risk for liver cancer as a result of the virus.

10. How can I determine whether I have chronic viral hepatitis, and what do I do if I have it?

Your doctor can perform blood tests to determine whether you have ever been exposed to hepatitis B and C in the past. If you have cleared the virus, then you are not contagious to others. Nevertheless, your family members should be tested because you were contagious during the acute viral infection.

The blood tests can also determine whether you have chronic hepatitis B or C. If you have chronic viral infection, then you are at risk for developing cirrhosis and/or liver cancer. Your family members should be tested. You should also take precautions so that you do not transmit the virus to your family. Medications can be taken to treat chronic hepatitis B or C infection. A liver specialist will determine whether you should be treated and with what drug. The goal of the treatment is to reduce the amount of virus in your body and thus lower the risk of getting cirrhosis or cancer. A liver **biopsy** may be performed to determine whether you have signs of liver damage now. For hepatitis B, the drugs that are used include **interferon-a, lamivudine**, and **adefovir**. Interferon-a and **ribavirin** are used for hepatitis C. You will

Risk Fac*

Biopsy

the physical sampling of a piece of tissue. In patients with a suspected tumor, a biopsy is used to determine whether the patient has a cancer and what type of tumor it is.

Interferon-α

a protein that is produced by specific cells in response to infection or cancer in an aim to protect the body. It is used to treat hepatitis.

Lamivudine

an antivirus drug that is commonly used against HIV and also against hepatitis C.

Adefovir

an antiviral drug that is used for patients with chronic hepatitis B.

Ribavirin

an antiviral drug.

also be advised to enter a screening program, as discussed later here. In many patients who develop liver cancer from chronic hepatitis, the cancer develops only after years of viral infection. For instance, cirrhosis can develop 10 years after exposure to hepatitis B, and then 10 years after that a tumor may form.

11. How does alcohol use affect my liver?

Alcohol use is another risk factor for liver cancer. **Alcoholic liver disease** is caused by chronic and excessive ingestion of alcohol. The quantity and duration of alcohol intake are the most important factors. An average of 60 to 80 grams of alcohol intake per day puts a person at high risk for developing liver disease. This amount is equivalent to an average of 6 cans of beer, 23 ounces of wine, or 6 ounces of 80% proof spirits. A smaller amount of alcohol ingestion in women can lead to cirrhosis and thus liver cancer. Another consequence of alcohol on the liver is the development of a **fatty liver**, which can occur in over 90% of heavy drinkers and binge drinkers.

Alcoholic liver disease
liver cirrhosis caused by excessive alcohol ingestion.

12. What are the inherited metabolic diseases that affect the liver?

Several rare inherited diseases can cause liver damage and may lead to cirrhosis and/or liver cancer. Two of these diseases lead to the accumulation of a mineral in the liver and result in cirrhosis, which increases the risk of liver cancer.

Hemochromatosis is an illness of increased iron absorption and deposition in many organs of the body, including the liver. The disease is inherited and is most commonly seen among northern Europeans or their descendants. People who are affected can live a normal

Fatty liver
condition in which fat accumulates in the liver because of a liver illness caused by one of several diseases (e.g., viral hepatitis).

Hemochromatosis
a hereditary disease that leads to excessive accumulation of iron in the body and may cause liver disease and ultimately primary liver cancer.

many (especially men) start to have symptoms he age of 40 years. Affected individuals may eel tired and weak and may acquire a shiny tan skin in the absence of sun exposure because of osition in the skin. People of northern Euro-nicity may know of family relatives who have ken from them very frequently. This is done to reduce the amount of iron in the body because blood contains a lot of iron. If you have the symptoms listed or have family members affected by this disease, you might need to be screened for hemochromatosis. The increased deposition of iron in the liver may lead to liver cirrhosis, liver failure, and cancer.

Wilson's disease

an inherited disease of impaired copper metabolism.

Wilson's disease is another genetic disease that pro-duces liver cancer. It causes the accumulation of copper throughout the body, including the liver. This inability to maintain a proper copper balance in the body is due to the lack of a protein called **ceruloplasmin**. Nor-mally, ceruloplasmin helps rid the body of excess cop-per. In its absence, a hepatitis inflammatory condition might occur, leading ultimately to cirrhosis and then liver cancer.

Ceruloplasmin

a protein that binds to copper.

Multiple other genetic diseases that might cause inflammation in the liver (hepatitis) and cirrhosis can also lead to the development of liver cancer. Some of these diseases are listed in Table 3.

Aflatoxins

a group of molds that contaminate stored food supplies and may lead to cirrhosis and ultimately liver cancer.

13. What environmental factors may cause liver cancer?

Exposure to **aflatoxins** is associated with liver cancer. Aflatoxins are produced by two **fungi** called *Aspergillus flavus* and *Aspergillus parasiticus*. These fungi usually grow

Fungus

a type of organism than can cause an infection.

Table 3 Genetic Diseases That May Cause Liver Cancer

Hemochromatosis
Wilson's disease
Alpha-1 antitrypsin deficiency
Primary biliary cirrhosis
Porphyria cutanea tarda
Types 1 and 3 glycogen storage disease
Galactosemia
Citrullinemia
Hereditary tyrosinemia
Familial cholestatic cirrhosis
Familial polyposis coli
Ataxia telangiectasia
Biliary atresia
Congenital hepatic fibrosis
Neurofibromatosis
Situs inversus
Fetal alcohol syndrome
Budd-Chiari syndrome

on grains, peanuts, and other food products. This is especially a hazard in certain African regions and in southern China. These fungi are responsible for most food spoilage in these tropical regions. Liver toxicity from aflatoxins may lead to the development of liver cancer.

Certain chemicals, such as nitrites, hydrocarbons, solvents, and organochlorine pesticides, may cause liver cancer. Your doctor and possibly an environmental health doctor need to evaluate you carefully if you have been exposed to these chemicals. Other factors may still need to be considered because a definitive relationship has not been proven for each type of chemical exposure.

14. Do obesity and diabetes cause liver cancer?

Obesity and type II diabetes are closely associated with a type of liver abnormality called **nonalcoholic fatty liver disease** that might lead to cirrhosis and ultimately liver cancer. This is an emerging concept that has not yet been proven. If you are obese or have diabetes, your doctor will discuss these potential risk factors and any precautions that should be taken.

Nonalcoholic fatty liver disease

disease that leads to the development of fatty liver by injuries other than excessive alcohol use.

15. How can I reduce my risk of getting liver cancer?

A number of things can be done to lower the risk of getting liver cancer. If you already have chronic hepatitis, then you should consult with your doctor about taking medication to help clear the virus from your body. You should also avoid behavior that may expose you to another type of hepatitis virus. For instance, if you have chronic hepatitis B, then try to avoid infection with hepatitis C. Having both chronic hepatitis B and C together substantially raises your risk of liver cirrhosis and liver cancer. Obviously, if you use excessive alcohol, seek medical help to try to treat your dependency. Also, excessive alcohol use should be avoided if you have chronic hepatitis. If you have an inherited disease that puts you at higher risk of liver cancer, work closely with your doctor to optimize the treatment of your condition. Patients who have concerns about environmental exposures should consult with an environmental medicine physician and possibly a liver specialist. Similarly, if you have diabetes or are severely obese, you should be under close medical attention.

PART THREE

Screening

Who should be screened for liver cancer?

Why is screening for liver cancer performed?

What does screening entail?

More . . .

16. Who should be screened for liver cancer?

From a practical standpoint, a person who carries any of the previously discussed risk factors should be potentially screened for liver cancer. For example, individuals with chronic hepatitis B or C infection should be regularly evaluated by a physician for the development of liver cirrhosis and liver cancer. This also applies to individuals with a history of excess alcohol ingestion, especially if they have liver problems; patients with a family history for any genetic disease that carries a risk of developing liver cancer; and patients with an environmental risk, especially if they already have evident liver problems. It is particularly important to mention that no specific guidelines exist regarding screening, and this should be carefully discussed with your physician to assess the benefits and risks of any screening studies that may be recommended. For example, screening is recommended for any patient who has chronic hepatitis B or C, but we do not necessarily recommend the same approach for individuals with exposure to certain chemicals or those who have other known liver problems.

17. Why is screening for liver cancer performed?

The reason to screen patients who are thought to be at high risk of developing a liver cancer is that if a liver cancer does occur, the tumor will more likely be detected at an early stage. Otherwise, many patients with liver cancer have advanced disease by the time they seek medical attention and the diagnosis is made. This happens for two reasons. First, the liver does not sense pain very well. Only the outside lining of the liver (called the **liver capsule**) has **nerve** fibers. Therefore, a tumor inside of the liver may not cause any symptoms of pain. Second, the liver has a tremendous functional reserve. As a result, even an advanced tumor may not alter the normal function of the liver and may not cause any abnormalities on routine blood work. In general, we recommend screening because we think that patients with early-stage liver tumors have the best chance of being cured of their disease. Nevertheless, the precise benefit of finding cancers when they are small has not been definitively proven.

18. What does screening entail?

This is a controversial issue; however, most physicians recommend an **ultrasound** of the liver and a blood test called **α-fetoprotein**, known as AFP.

An ultrasound uses sound waves to image internal organs. This is the same test that is used to look at fetuses in pregnant women. During an ultrasound of the liver, a technician or doctor places a probe over your liver, which is located in the upper right portion of your abdomen. The test is typically easy and painless and does not involve any injections or **radiation** exposure. You may feel some pressure at the site being evaluated as the probe is pushed close to your body. Some doctors may prefer to use a different type of radiologic test such as a **computed tomography** (CT) scan or a **magnetic resonance imaging** (MRI), both of which are described in Question 23.

AFP is a protein that appears in the blood of approximately 80% of patients with liver cancer. Therefore, a positive blood test for AFP can be an early indicator

Liver capsule

the outside lining of the liver. It is the only part of the liver that can trigger a sensation of pain.

Nerve

a type of tissue in the body that can transmit sensations such as pain, pressure, or temperature.

Ultrasound

the use of ultrasonic waves to view images of an internal body structure.

α-Fetoprotein

a blood marker that may be elevated in primary liver cancer.

Radiation

a ray of powerful energy that is emitted from a radioactive material.

Computed tomography (CT scan)

a form of x-ray images in which acquired images are constructed by computer to form cross-sectional images of the body.

Magnetic resonance imaging (MRI)

a form of radiologic imaging that uses magnetic fields to produce electronic images of the inner parts of the human body.

that a patient has a liver cancer. However, AFP alone is insufficient as a screening tool, as certain liver cancers do not secrete or produce AFP. Thus, a normal AFP level could be misleading. Also, not every elevated AFP level implies the presence of liver cancer. Many other situations exist where AFP can be elevated. For example, it is normally elevated in pregnancy. AFP can also be elevated in other cancers such as testicular cancer and stomach cancer. Screening for liver cancer relies on a comprehensive assessment and evaluation conducted by your physician and does not rely on any single test.

19. How often should a patient who is at high risk of liver cancer be screened?

This unsettled issue is currently being studied. No universal consensus of opinion is available at this time. At the Memorial Sloan-Kettering Cancer Center, we recommend that a liver specialist evaluate patients who are at high risk of developing liver cancer every 3 to 6 months. We generally recommend liver blood tests and an AFP level and a liver ultrasound.

20. What should be done if a screening test suggests that a patient has a liver cancer?

If an ultrasound shows or suggests a liver mass and/or if the AFP is elevated, further tests will be required. A CT scan or an MRI is often used to evaluate abnormal ultrasound findings or an elevated AFP. If an abnormality is confirmed, you should be evaluated by a multidisciplinary group of doctors and other health care professionals, as discussed in Questions 29 and 34.

PART FOUR

Diagnosis and Staging

What are the symptoms of liver cancer?

Are the symptoms of liver cancer different in a patient with cirrhosis?

How is liver cancer diagnosed?

More ...

21. What are the symptoms of liver cancer?

As discussed in Question 17, by the time a liver cancer causes symptoms, many patients already have advanced disease. The most common symptom is a dull abdominal ache below the right rib cage, where the liver is located. The pain may sometimes travel to the right shoulder. Patients might lose weight or have a fever that is not explained by any infection. On physical examination, your doctor might detect that your liver is enlarged or even feel a mass in the liver. Some patients have no symptoms, and a tumor is detected on screening tests or during blood work or radiologic tests performed to evaluate other conditions.

22. Are the symptoms of liver cancer different in a patient with cirrhosis?

In many instances, cirrhosis is the breeding ground for the development of liver cancer. Many times liver cancer can present as worsening cirrhosis. The liver as a large organ can compensate for cirrhosis, the causes of which are discussed previously. However, sometimes the cirrhosis worsens, and the liver fails. One reason for this liver failure is that as the liver tumor replaces the noncancerous liver, which is already abnormal from cirrhosis, the patient has no further reserve of liver function. In this case, a liver tumor may cause worsening cirrhosis.

Abdominal distention

bulging of the belly.

Ascites

an abnormal accumulation of fluid in the abdomen.

Peripheral edema

excessive accumulation of fluids in the legs that leads to swelling.

Several things normally occur in cirrhosis, any of which can be worsened by a liver tumor (Table 4). A patient may have **abdominal distention**, with fluid buildup in the abdomen, called **ascites**. Fluid buildup can also occur in the legs and is called **peripheral edema**. Patients may also acquire a yellowish discol-

Table 4   Complications of Cirrhosis

Ascites
Peripheral edema
Jaundice
Mental confusion
Portal hypertension
Variceal bleeding

oration to their skin and eyes, called jaundice. Jaundice also results in a lighter color of stools because bile is not released into the intestine to give stool its normal dark color. Because the pigments in bile cannot be processed by the liver in jaundice, they are excreted by the **kidneys**, resulting in dark or tea-colored urine. Further decompensation of the liver might lead to its inability to metabolize or get rid of different toxins. These may accumulate in the body, including the brain, and may cause mental confusion, drowsiness, or sleepiness, called **encephalopathy**. This decompensation associated with liver cancer growth can also be explained by the possible direct growth of the cancer into the blood supply of the liver. Clogged vessels near the tumor might build up pressure on the vessels on the outside of the liver. This is called **portal hypertension**. This buildup of pressure could lead to abnormally swollen or dilated small vessels that ultimately may break and bleed. A typical place for this bleeding to occur is in the stomach or esophagus. A patient might experience bloody or dark vomiting or might notice tarry stools. Sometimes the patients may not notice the bleeding but will become tired. These **variceal bleeds** warrant immediate medical evaluation.

Kidneys
two organs located in the abdomen that are responsible for water and electrolytes balance, and that help excrete body metabolites through urine.

Encephalopathy
an altered sense of consciousness. It may occur when the liver is not working well.

Portal hypertension
increased pressure within the veins of the liver.

Variceal bleed
an actively bleeding varix, which is a dilated vein.

23. How is liver cancer diagnosed?

If a patient is suspected of having a liver tumor based on screening tests or experiences new symptoms, he or she will require a more definitive imaging test, such as a CT scan or an MRI. A CT scan is a computer-generated picture of multiple x-rays of the body taken at different angles—the collection of which make up sliced pictures of the human body. An MRI makes a similar picture but uses a magnetic field instead of radiation. Although MRIs sound more appealing because they do not require radiation, the amount of radiation exposure during a CT scan is not dangerous. A patient who is claustrophobic may have difficulty with an MRI because he or she will have to lie still in a confined tube during the test. Patients who have certain metal parts in their body, such as an artificial knee, may not be eligible for an MRI. Usually a patient is given a questionnaire to determine whether he or she can obtain an MRI. MRIs are still not widely available, and because CT scans have been performed for a much longer time, some **radiologists** might have more experience reading them than an MRI. The doctor knows which test is better for a patient, as each may provide slightly different information. A mass or multiple masses in the liver might be noted. It is important to mention that liver cancer can invade local blood vessels and block them. It also can invade local **lymph nodes** or even spread to other organs. A good imaging study should usually identify these possibilities. Three general growth patterns of hepatocellular cancer exist inside the liver. The tumor can grow as a well-circumscribed nodule. The tumor can be more invasive and grow diffusely without any apparent boundaries in an

Radiologists

doctors who specialize in interpreting x-rays, CTs, MRIs, and other radiologic tests.

Lymph nodes

small bodies along the lymphatic system that supply a special kind of fighter white blood cells called lymphocytes to the bloodstream.

area of the liver. Hepatocellular cancer can also grow as multiple nodules scattered within the liver.

An AFP blood test will be obtained if it has not been already performed. Although an elevated AFP (normal is usually 0 to 15 ng/ml) may suggest the presence of liver cancer, it is nonspecific and may reflect another medical condition in the body. More importantly, some liver cancers do not cause an elevated AFP. Thus, this test by itself is not diagnostic but is complementary to multiple other radiologic and blood tests that your doctor might ask for. An elevation of AFP above 400 mg/dl is considered virtually diagnostic of a liver cancer in the appropriate clinical setting. The degree of AFP elevation does not necessarily reflect the amount of disease present because even small tumors can produce substantial amounts of the protein.

Despite how advanced the technology seems, CT and MRI scans are not always ultra-precise. Depending on the exact machine and the skill of the operator, the scans can sometimes be fuzzy and subject to interpretation. For example, the CT scan report may show that the tumor measures 3.2 by 1.8 mm one month and then 3.4 mm by 1.9 mm just a couple of weeks later. However, depending on where that measurement was taken, that may or may not indicate the tumor has really grown. Also, sometimes small spots or lesions can show up on the scan that may or may not be cancerous or related. We would always try to ask the radiologist for copies of the report and then ask the doctor for his best educated guess and interpretation of progress relative to the previous report.

24. Is a biopsy required for diagnosis?

As with most other cancers, the ultimate proof that you have a cancer depends on a biopsy, which is performed by sampling a piece of the tumor. In some instances, a surgeon might elect to remove a tumor without obtaining a biopsy of the tumor. This decision would be built on a collection of evidence to proceed directly to surgery without first obtaining a biopsy. For instance, if you have an AFP of greater than 400 mg/dl and a mass that is consistent with a hepatocellular cancer on a CT or an MRI, then a biopsy may not be required. In other instances, your doctor may require a biopsy. Most **oncologists** require a biopsy before starting **chemotherapy** to treat a cancer.

A biopsy of a liver tumor is typically obtained via a needle that is placed through the skin. To ensure the safety and adequacy of the sample, a needle biopsy is usually performed under radiologic guidance using either an ultrasound or a CT scan. The procedure itself is relatively safe and causes only minor discomfort. A **local anesthetic** will be injected into your skin to minimize any pain. The doctor performing the procedure will discuss the potential complications of a biopsy. These are rare. They include the possibility of bleeding or infection.

25. What is a pathology report of a biopsy?

The tissue obtained by a biopsy is typically sent to a **pathology laboratory**, where is it sliced into very thin cuts that are applied to 3 × 1-inch glass slides, known as **pathology slides**. The very thin cuts are stained with different chemicals that color various structures. A **pathologist** then looks at these under a microscope.

Oncologists

medical doctor specialists who treat cancer.

Chemotherapy

chemical agents that are used to treat cancer.

Local anesthetic

numbing medication that is injected directly at the site where a procedure is to be performed.

Pathology laboratory

the section of the hospital in which a pathologist works and where tissue specimens are analyzed.

Pathology slides

3 × 1 inch glass slides on which tissue from a biopsy or a surgical specimen is placed.

Pathologist

a doctor who specializes in the diagnosis of diseases of the body.

A pathologist can view the cancerous cells and estimate how aggressive they are. Because many cancers can metastasize the liver, the pathologist also needs to confirm that the tumor is indeed hepatocellular cancer and not another primary liver cancer or a secondary liver cancer. Based on the findings of the pathologist, a typed **pathology report** is generated.

26. What is cancer staging, and why is it relevant?

Patients and physicians alike need a way to communicate the status of a cancer. Liver cancer can involve one or more sites in the liver, blood vessels in and around the liver, lymph nodes close to the liver and distant organs such as bone. To be able to communicate this information and decide on a plan of care, physicians use a **staging system**. In liver cancer, the first step in staging a tumor is to determine whether it consists of one or more tumors, its size or sizes, whether it involves any blood vessels, and whether it has any further local extension. This is given a T (for tumor) score. Lymph nodes are evaluated next and are given an N (for node) score, and finally, any disease that has spread to other sites is given an M (for metastasis) score. Combining the T, N, and M scores assigns a stage to the cancer that ranges between I and IV. Stages I and II indicate a tumor that is confined to the liver. Stage III is subdivided into groups A, B, or C and includes cancers that invade major blood vessels, other organs in close proximity to the liver, or lymph nodes. Stage IV disease is any disease that has spread beyond the liver or the region of the liver.

Pathology report

a typed report issued by a pathologist that describes the results of the analysis of a biopsy or surgical specimen.

Staging system

a set of definitions that allows physicians to define the extent of a certain cancer and recommend therapy accordingly.

PART FIVE

Coping with the Diagnosis

How long do people live with liver cancer?

Does cirrhosis influence the treatment of liver cancer and the quality and length of life?

What is multidisciplinary care?

More ...

27. How long do people live with liver cancer?

This is a difficult question, and no simple answer is available. How someone will do depends on the stage of his or her cancer, his or her general medical condition, the health of the part of his or her liver not affected by cancer, and the treatment options that he or she is eligible for. Your doctor can give you an idea of how you may do. However, even experienced physicians often cannot accurately determine how one particular patient may fare. Building a close relationship with your physicians is important to help deal with your fears that might build up after being diagnosed with cancer. Your doctors should be in a position to recommend the best approach of therapy based on the stage of the disease. This, by itself, might influence the possibility of cure and survival.

28. Does cirrhosis influence the treatment of liver cancer and the quality and length of life?

In contrast to many other cancers, liver cancer is often two diseases in one. Cirrhosis by itself contributes to the development of cancer and directly affects the level of function of the liver. A cirrhotic liver will be unable to synthesize or make the essential required proteins and bile. It will also fail to metabolize or break down the different compounds that go through the liver. A badly cirrhotic liver can actually be a worse problem than the cancer it harbors and might affect survival. Even therapeutic decisions regarding the cancer might be influenced by the degree of cirrhosis. Although a cancer specialist may treat a patient with primary liver cancer, often a liver specialist (**hepatologist**) should also be involved. Cirrhosis is graded using different criteria. One of the more commonly used grading systems is the **Child Pugh score**. This score assesses the synthetic and metabolic functions of the liver. The score ranges between A and C, with C being the worst.

Hepatologist
a liver disease specialist.

Child Pugh score
a score used to assess the level of cirrhosis.

29. What is multidisciplinary care?

The diagnosis of liver cancer may have a severe impact on a patient. In addition to the cancer itself and, if present, cirrhosis, other concerns, including nutrition and pain control, might be present. This is not to understate the psychologic social and financial impact. A person who is working and is found to have liver cancer might have his or her life come to a halt. As much as this might seem very discouraging, we believe that a multidisciplinary team approach might alleviate many, if not all, of these concerns. In addition to a variety of doctors (see Question 34), you may also need the help of pain specialists, nutritionists, psychiatrists, and social workers. A typical comprehensive cancer center has a team of several types of doctors and health care workers. In addition, patient support groups and **integrative medicine** may be helpful. Integrative medicine is a growing discipline that addresses the emotional, social, and spiritual needs of patients and their families. This helps to increase self-awareness and enhances well-being.

Integrative medicine
a discipline that is used to treat patients using modern science and alternative medicine.

30. Should a patient get a second opinion?

Patients who are diagnosed with cancer often obtain a second opinion. We do encourage second opinions, as they may provide the patient with more information. Of course, different doctors may have

Coping with the Diagnosis

different amounts of experience with liver cancer patients. As a result, you may actually receive conflicting opinions about what you should do. Patients should try to avoid getting too many opinions that may make things more confusing or even delay critical therapy. At initial diagnosis, seeking a second opinion could be very valuable, as certain therapeutic options, such as surgery or liver transplantation, may not be available locally and a patient may need to seek medical care at a larger cancer center. In patients with very advanced disease, the need for a second opinion is less critical. Some patients and their families might take the challenge of traveling distances to seek opinions and look for miracles. In this instance, we recommend using common sense and good judgment to determine the need for such second opinions. More importantly, you need to have a frank and open discussion with your physician, who is in the right position to assess the usefulness of a second opinion. Do not be surprised if your physician is the one who suggests a second opinion. In either instance, this is not a reflection on the inability of your physician to handle the current medical situation but is rather a genuine effort to make you feel comfortable with the treatment that you will choose.

31. How should I manage my emotions now that I have been diagnosed with liver cancer?

People differ in the way that they react to any adverse event in life. Some patients might be geared emotionally to handle their new diagnosis with liver cancer and react positively, but others might see themselves facing difficult times as they deal with new emotions, feelings, and stress. Patients are not expected to understand their illness or to identify priorities immediately.

Accepting the diagnosis of cancer might take a while, as patients have to first deal with their fear, denial, and anger. Patients fear cancer in general because of the unknown and the uncertainty that it carries. Patients are encouraged to discuss this fear with their doctors, as the more they learn about their disease, the more they will feel in control of the situation and know better how to deal with the bad news. Patients might react with denial and anger, and it is better to circumvent those as well. Patients might direct their anger against other people. It is a very delicate situation, especially if people close to the patient, such as family members, are also angry. Patients and their loved ones are encouraged to spell out their fears and angers and to realize that they are facing the same situation and that they need each other's help.

Guilt might also be present, especially because some of the causes of liver cancer listed previously here result from a person's lifestyle, such as using shared needles for intravenous drug use and consuming alcohol. Guilt is normal and is best dealt with by accepting the current condition. Some patients might start building positively on the current situation. One of our patients, realizing the consequences of his previous use of intravenous drugs, is now a licensed counselor who helps others.

The other common emotion of a cancer patient is **depression**, which is again a normal and expected reaction to the acceptance of the new diagnosis of liver cancer. Patients should be aware of its signs and symptoms, as many of them can be confounded with those

Depression
a sad state of mind characterized by feeling tired, with an inability to concentrate, an inability to sleep, a decreased appetite, guilt, and thoughts of death.

symptoms of the cancer itself, such as a loss of appetite and a decreased level of energy. Nonetheless, even the subtle feeling of being depressed should be shared with the physician so that corrective action can be taken.

Patients are encouraged to have an open discussion with their caregivers about any concerns. In many instances, professional help from a psychiatrist or even medications might be needed, and this should be accepted as part of the healing process.

32. What insurance and financial concerns does a patient need to address after a diagnosis of liver cancer?

This is an important aspect of medical care nowadays. Health care is expensive, and patients with liver cancer might need to stop working, at least temporarily. This might affect their insurance coverage. After being diagnosed with liver cancer, you need to start collecting information about the health coverage options that you have. Does the health insurance company provide only in-network coverage, thus making a patient select from the different providers and/or hospitals with which his or her insurance company has an agreement? Is there out-of-network coverage that allows a patient to seek medical care where he or she may wish? All individuals should make sure that all of their insurance premiums are paid and that all information is up-to-date. Patients should make sure to document all contacts with their insurance company. Organized and well-documented information might save a lot of trouble later on. Most hospitals have a patient financial services department. It is important to establish contact with such a department to understand your rights and obligations.

Based on the severity of the illness or the extent of the treatment prescribed, patients might be required to take a sick leave or even be placed on disability. This can be done through a workplace or private insurance disability policy that may already be in place.

The government also has many programs that may help you. These are divided into two big categories. Programs that are not based on income or financial means include Medicare for patients above 65 years of age. Details about the program may be found on the official website: *www.medicare.gov*. Another is social security (*www.ssa.gov*) for patients above 65 years of age and social security disability (*www.ssa.gov*) for disabled workers and their family based on disabled status and their prior contribution to the program. U.S. Veterans might also seek veterans' benefits through the Veterans Affairs Department.

If a patient does not have the means to obtain health care, he or she may seek government support through Medicaid. Details about the program can be found at *http://cms.hhs.gov/medicaid*.

PART SIX

Treatment

What treatment options are available for liver cancer?

Who decides what therapy I should receive?

What determines whether a tumor can be removed?

More . . .

33. What treatment options are available for liver cancer?

Several treatment options are available for patients with hepatocellular carcinoma (Table 5). In the majority of patients, the liver cancer has not spread outside the liver at the time of diagnosis. In general, for these patients, the most effective therapy is to remove the tumor. This can be done in two ways. One method is to remove the part of the liver that contains the tumor. This is called **liver resection** or **partial hepatectomy**. The other option is to remove your entire liver and replace it with a new liver. This is called liver transplantation.

If the tumor cannot be removed, then doctors may recommend that it be ablated. **Ablation** means to kill as much of the tumor as possible without removing it. There are four principal techniques. **Hepatic artery embolization** is a procedure in which the blood vessels of your tumor are clogged by injecting them with a substance. **Alcohol injection** is performed by injecting alcohol directly into the tumor. **Radiofrequency abla-**

Liver resection
the surgical removal of all or a portion of the liver.

Partial hepatectomy
the surgical removal of part of the liver.

Ablation
the destruction of a tumor without actually removing it.

Hepatic artery embolization
the injection of microscopic particles (either attached to a chemotherapy drug or not) into the branches of the hepatic artery in order to ablate or destroy a liver tumor.

Alcohol injection
inserting alcohol through a needle into a tumor.

Table 5   Treatments For Hepatocellular Cancer

Liver resection
Liver transplantation
Hepatic artery embolization
Radiofrequency ablation
Alcohol injection
Cryotherapy
Chemotherapy
Investigational chemotherapy
Biologic and targeted therapy
Supportive care
Investigational biologic or targeted therapy

tion (also known as RFA) is done by inserting a metal probe into the tumor to then heat it up in order to kill the cancer cells. **Cryotherapy** is performed with a metal probe that freezes the tumor. Chemotherapy is the use of drugs to kill your liver tumor. It may involve standard drugs or new agents that are under investigation. Each of these treatments is discussed in detail later.

34. Who decides what therapy I should receive?

A team of doctors will help you decide which treatment to pursue. Each of these doctors has a different area of expertise, and together they can make the best recommendations. A **hepatobiliary surgeon** is a specialist in liver surgery and will decide whether your tumor can be removed. A patient may be referred to a liver transplant surgeon if liver transplantation is a consideration. A medical oncologist is a cancer specialist that specializes in the use of chemotherapy, biologic therapy, and other nonsurgical treatments of liver cancer. A hepatologist is a doctor that specifically deals with liver diseases that might have caused liver cancer or cirrhosis. A hepatologist also treats the complications caused by cirrhosis and the cancer itself.

Immediately after my father was diagnosed in 2000, the doctors recommended that he undergo resection to remove the single tumor in his liver. This course of action offered the best hope of a complete cure. His general health was very good, and the tumor was isolated in the left lobe of his liver. Much to our chagrin, though, the hepatobiliary surgeon decided, after closer investigation, that his liver was too cirrhotic and that recovery from resection would be too risky.

Radiofrequency ablation

a form of tumor ablation that relies on heating to destroy tumor cells.

Cryotherapy

a form of therapy that uses cold temperature to kill cancer cells.

Hepatobiliary surgeon

a doctor who specializes in the surgical and ablative treatments of liver, gallbladder, bile duct, and pancreas tumors.

Treatment

Therefore, over the next 4 years, his doctors focused on managing the tumor(s) by a combination of alcohol (ethanol) injections and embolizations. This regimen worked well for my father and preserved a good quality of life for him.

35. What determines whether a tumor can be removed?

Several factors determine whether a liver tumor can be removed. These include (1) your health, (2) the condition of the portion of your liver without tumor, and (3) the distribution of the cancer and its relationship to vital structures of the liver.

Anesthesia

medication that puts someone to sleep and/or reduces pain.

First, the patient must be in adequate general health in order to tolerate general **anesthesia** and a major operation such as liver resection. For instance, if a patient has a weak heart, an attempt at a liver resection may not be advisable because it may be too dangerous.

The noncancerous part of your liver must be healthy enough in order to undergo a liver resection. The liver is a unique organ because it can regrow after part of it is removed. The liver is divided into right and left lobes, and it is composed of a total of eight individual segments. Up to six segments of a healthy liver can be removed in some patients. Remarkably, the liver regrows within about 2 weeks after resection. Normal liver function is restored within 4 weeks of a liver resection. If the liver is healthy, up to about 80% of it can be removed safely. However, many patients with hepatocellular cancer have cirrhosis of the liver (discussed previously), and thus, often only a smaller percentage of liver can be safely removed. Most patients with advanced cirrhosis cannot undergo liver resection because they have a high chance of dying from the operation. They can die from bleeding that occurs during or shortly after the operation because patients with advanced cirrhosis have difficulty in forming a blood clot. They can also die from liver failure in the first few weeks after liver resection. Their liver may function well enough for everyday living, but it may not handle the stress of a liver resection.

There are additional surgical factors relating to the extent of the cancer within the liver and its relationship to the vital structures of the liver. Most patients who are treated with liver resection have a single tumor. Sometimes patients with two or three tumors will also be treated with liver resection. Patients with more than three tumors are usually not offered resection as an option because it is less beneficial to them. The vital structures of the liver include the bile duct, which carries bile out of the liver, and the blood vessels. Blood is brought into the liver via the **hepatic artery** and the **portal vein**. The bile duct, hepatic artery, and portal vein branch into left and right branches, which in turn branch many more times. Blood is removed from the liver via the three hepatic veins. A large vein, called the **inferior vena cava**, is behind the liver and gets blood from the hepatic veins and also directly from small branches from the liver that drain directly into it. The inferior vena cava also returns all of the blood from the lower half of your body to the heart. At the end of a liver resection, the patient must have an intact bile duct, portal vein, and hepatic artery supply and hepatic vein drainage of the liver (Figure 2).

Hepatic artery

the blood vessel that carries oxygenated blood to the liver.

Portal vein

a blood vessel that carries blood from the intestines to within the liver.

Inferior vena cava

a large vein that is supplied by multiple veins from the lower parts of the body and helps bring the blood back to the heart.

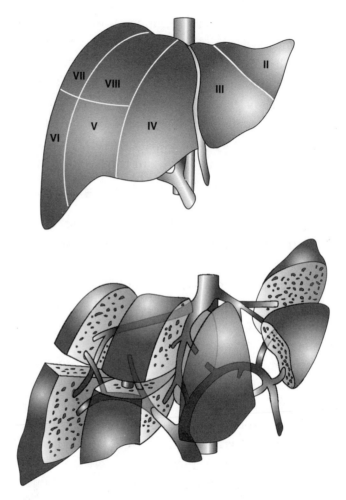

Figure 2   The liver is made up of 8 segments, each with its own blood supply, blood drainage, and bile drainage. Reprinted by permission of Memorial Sloan-Kettering Cancer Center.

36. What preparations are made before a liver resection?

After the patient and doctor decide that a liver resection should be attempted, certain preparations will be made. If the patient is older or has certain medical problems, he or she may need to see a general medicine doctor or a cardiologist to determine whether he or she is fit enough for an operation. He or she may even be asked to undergo certain special tests. For instance, a patient may be given a stress test or **echocardiogram** to evaluate his or her heart function.

Next, the patient will get what is called "preadmission testing." This includes routine blood tests, an **electrocardiogram**, and a chest x-ray. This is standard practice before undergoing general anesthesia. Often the patient will also meet with an **anesthesiologist**. In most cases, patients will be admitted the day of the operation. If special medical circumstances exist, a patient may be admitted to the hospital 1 day or a few days before the operation. Depending on the location of the tumor, the surgeon may have the patient undergo a colon preparation using some medication to clean out the intestines before surgery.

On the morning of surgery, the patient is not allowed to eat or drink. The physician will have told you whether to take your normal medications with a sip of water. You will be asked to arrive at the hospital several hours before the scheduled time of the operation. You may be asked to arrive as early as 6 a.m. because most surgeons start early in the morning. You will be asked to get undressed and to put on a hospital gown. Patients will generally be kept in a holding area until the operating room is ready. In some hospitals, families may be able to stay with the patient at that time. Many staff members will likely ask you your name, your medical history, the intended surgical procedure, and your allergies. Such repetition may become annoying but is done to ensure your safety.

Echocardiogram

a test for the heart in which pictures and functional values of the heart are obtained using ultrasound.

Electrocardiogram

an electrical tracing of the heart.

Anesthesiologist

a doctor who specializes in the delivery of anesthesia.

Ultimately, the patient is taken into the operating room. This is usually done using a wheelchair. The patient will meet several nurses, surgical assistants, an anesthesiologist, and the surgeon. The operating room is often somewhat cold, but you will be covered with several blankets during the operation. An intravenous (IV) will be started in the arm if it was not placed already in the holding area. You will be placed flat on a table and asked to breathe through a mask and will then be put to sleep.

37. What happens during a liver resection?

After you are asleep, the hair that is on your belly (if you have any) will be shaved, and your belly will be washed with soap. Generally, a small tube, called a **Foley catheter**, will be placed into the bladder so that the amount of urine can be closely monitored. A larger IV may be placed into the neck to give more fluids and/or medications that might be needed for support through the operation.

In some circumstances, the surgeon may decide to perform a **laparoscopy** immediately before your liver resection or sometime beforehand. A laparoscopy is performed with the patient under general anesthesia. A few small incisions (less than an inch) are made in order to insert a telescope and some instruments in order to inspect the belly. Specifically, the surgeon is looking to see whether the cancer is more advanced than what is shown on the radiologic tests. If you have cirrhosis, the surgeon also determines whether your cirrhosis is too advanced for you to undergo an operation safely.

A number of different incisions can be made to expose the liver during an open operation. The three most common are shown in Figure 3. Your surgeon will

Foley catheter

a tube that is placed into the bladder to monitor precisely the urine output of a patient.

Laparoscopy

a procedure that is done under general anesthesia and performed by a surgeon in which the inside of the abdomen can be examined through a few small incisions.

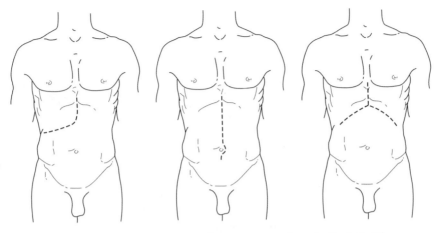

Figure 3   The 3 most common incisions for liver surgery are shown by the dotted lines. Reprinted by permission of Memorial Sloan-Kettering Cancer Center.

decide whether your tumor can be removed. Although your tumor may appear to be removable on a CT scan or MRI, the surgeon may find that your tumor cannot be removed because of any one of several findings:

1. The tumor has spread to the outside of the liver.
2. The tumor has spread to other areas within your liver.
3. The tumor cannot be safely removed from vital structures.
4. There is more advanced cirrhosis than anticipated.

If the tumor is removable, the surgeon will then proceed with liver resection. As part of the operation, the surgeon may have to remove your gallbladder to expose other structures of the liver. The gallbladder is a small organ that is situated on the edge of your liver. It functions as a storage tank for bile. Bile is stored in the gallbladder and is emptied into the intestine after we eat a meal. Basically, it helps you digest a large fatty meal. Patients can live a perfectly normal life without a gallbladder. In fact, removing the gallbladder for other reasons is one of the most common operations in the United States.

38. What happens in the hospital after a liver resection?

After the operation, you will be taken to a recovery room for close observation. The main risk within the first 12 hours is bleeding from the cut surface of the liver. Rarely, a patient needs to undergo an emergency operation to control bleeding. Depending on the hospital, you will stay in a highly monitored setting for 1 to 5 days and then be transferred to a regular patient floor. Overall, you can expect to be in the hospital between 5 and 10 days. If everything goes well, you should be able to sit in a chair and, in many cases, walk the day after your surgery. It often takes a few days before you are ready to eat again. A special intravenous pump that you control provides pain medication. The nurse will explain how to use it.

39. What are the risks of a liver resection?

Other potential complications of liver resection exist besides bleeding. Many patients will temporarily gain weight from the extra fluids that are given around the time of the operation. You may notice that your ankles are swollen from this. In some patients, the incision may not heal completely and actually separate slightly. This will require dressing changes while you are in the hospital and perhaps also when you are at home. About 10% of the time, a fluid collection will form where the liver was removed, and it will require drainage about a week later. This is usually done by having an **interven-**

tional radiologist insert a needle or a small drain into the collection. Other complications include infection in your urine because of the temporary tube that was placed into the bladder or **pneumonia.**

Patients with cirrhosis are at an additional risk of complications from an operation. They may develop gastrointestinal bleeding, which may arise from **gastritis** (stomach irritation), an **ulcer**, or **varices.** Varices are dilated veins in the esophagus or stomach. The veins dilate because the pressure within a cirrhotic liver is higher than normal. Patients with cirrhosis are also at risk for ascites, which is the accumulation of fluid within the belly. Ascites is generally treated with **diuretics** ("water pills") that make you urinate more frequently.

After you go home, complete recovery will take place over the next 3 to 6 weeks. You will slowly regain your energy. You may not notice that you are improving each day, but each week you will likely feel better. If you are not, then you should notify your doctor. Usually, if your doctor agrees, you can drive in a few weeks. You should not do any heavy lifting for several months so that you do not disrupt the incision. You should regain your quality of life in almost all cases.

40. What is included in the pathology report from my surgery?

The pathology report from your liver resection contains a lot of information. From it the precise stage of the cancer can be determined. The written report will state the size and number of the tumors. If lymph nodes were removed, the report will state whether

Treatment

Interventional radiologist

a doctor who specializes in performing procedures under radiologic (ultrasound, x-ray, or CT scan) guidance such as tumor biopsies and hepatic artery embolization.

Pneumonia

a lung infection.

Gastritis

inflammation of the inside lining of the stomach.

Ulcer

a lesion of the stomach that results from inflammation and may bleed.

Varix

an abnormally swollen vein that is prone to bleed.

Diuretics (water pills)

drugs that increase the discharge of urine.

tumor cells existed in them. Unlike many other cancers that are removed, in hepatocellular cancer, surgeons generally remove only the lymph nodes around the liver if they think that the nodes contain cancer. This is because most patients undergoing liver resections for hepatocellular cancer do not have involved nodes. Also, most surgeons will not remove the liver if lymph nodes are involved because, in general, the benefit of the operation is less. The pathologist also determines whether the surgeon achieved a negative margin of resection by entirely removing the tumor with a rim of normal tissue as a margin. The pathologist also dissects the liver and looks at the tumor under the microscope to determine whether the tumor invaded any large or small blood vessels. Patients with vascular invasion have a higher rate of having their tumor return in the future. The last piece of information is the status of the noncancerous liver. In other words, the pathologist will determine whether the liver has any signs of damage or cirrhosis.

41. Will I be cured after a liver resection?

In general, no one can predict whether your liver tumor will return after it is removed. Some patients are truly cured, meaning that their tumor never returns. Many patients, however, will have their tumor return at some point. If you have liver cirrhosis, you are also at risk of developing a new tumor. This happens for the same reasons that led to your original tumor. Thus, you should be followed carefully after your liver operation. If your blood level of AFP was elevated before the operation, then it is a good marker of whether your tumor has returned. It should be measured two to three times per year. The other primary method of surveillance after an operation is a CT, an MRI, or an ultrasound of your abdomen. These are often done two to four times per year for the first few years.

Doctors normally measure the outcome of patients with cancer by determining what percentage will be alive at 5 years. Again, it is important to stress that doctors generally cannot reliably predict what will happen to any given patient. It is like grades in school. The average grade in a class may be a "C"; however, some patients do a lot better, and others do a lot worse. In patients who undergo removal of a hepatocellular carcinoma, approximately 40% will still be alive 5 years later.

42. Should I receive adjuvant chemotherapy after liver resection to prevent recurrence of the tumor?

Adjuvant therapy is the use of chemotherapy, radiation, or any other form of treatment that is given after a cancer is surgically removed. In some other types of cancer, chemotherapy is routinely given after surgical removal of the tumor. It is done in an effort to kill any microscopic cells of cancer that might remain and thus prevent the recurrence of the cancer. However, at this time, the standard of care after the removal of hepatocellular carcinoma is just to observe the patient. Chemotherapy has not been proven to be beneficial enough to give after the tumor is removed. Of course, some **clinical trials** test new chemotherapy regimens or new agents that may improve the results of surgery. The key to improving long-term survival after liver resection is the development of more effective chemotherapy.

Adjuvant therapy
a form of therapy that will help prevent the recurrence of cancer after a potentially curative treatment such as surgery.

Clinical trial
a research study that answers many of the questions regarding newly discovered therapies.

43. Are other methods available to prevent the return of the cancer after a curative surgery?

One clinical trial of adjuvant therapy suggested its benefit after the removal of a hepatocellular cancer. Investigators from Hong Kong found that patients who were randomized to **radioactive lipiodol embolization** within 6 weeks of their surgery fared better than those who did not. Lipiodol is an inert substance, and during the trial it was attached to radioactive iodine. The compound was delivered into the hepatic artery of the liver via the leg artery. Although promising, this clinical trial was very small, and the results have never been repeated, making the true value of this approach uncertain. This therapy is not approved in the United States, and neither are any other adjuvant therapies for hepatocellular cancer. Other methods of prevention of recurrence that have been tested include interferon, which is known to have anticancer activity. This, however, failed to show any advantage from this perspective. It is discussed in Question 44 as a suppressor of the hepatitis virus, which is a cause of the cancer. Many other substances have been tested, including retinoic acid (Vitamin A) and **somatostatin analogues**; however, thus far, they have all lacked efficacy in large phase III trials.

44. If the tumor cannot be resected now, can I have chemotherapy first and then go to surgery?

Chemotherapy that is given before surgery in order to shrink the tumor and to allow it to be resected is called **neoadjuvant therapy**. As with adjuvant therapy, no

Radioactive lipiodol embolization

a procedure in which the blood vessels of the liver tumor are clogged by injecting them with the inert substance lipiodol that is tagged to radioactive material as an additional form of therapy.

Somatostatin analogues

variants of a hormonal protein that may be used to prevent the recurrence of primary liver cancer.

Neoadjuvant therapy

therapy that is given before surgical removal of a cancer, aiming at reducing its size and rendering it more resectable.

established standard of care is available for neoadjuvant treatment. The best data come from a limited study that was performed at the Chinese University of Hong Kong where 50 patients were tried on a combination of three chemotherapy drugs (cisplatin, doxorubicin, and 5-fluorouracil) and interferon (an immune booster)—known as PIAF (see Question 64). Of the 50 patients, 13 had a major response to therapy, and of the 13, 9 went back to surgery and had their tumor resected. Although this approach is not established as a standard of care, it can undoubtedly be used if it seems feasible based on a discussion among the patient, surgeon, and medical oncologist.

45. What happens if my tumor returns?

Your doctor may discover that your tumor has returned based on the serum AFP level, radiologic tests, or new symptoms that you are having. Several options are available if your tumor returns. Approximately 10% of the time, you may be eligible for another liver resection. Reoperation depends on the same factors listed in Question 35 and the extent of the first liver operation. The other treatment options include all of those listed later for initially unresectable tumors—liver transplantation, tumor ablation, chemotherapy, or supportive care.

46. Why is liver transplantation performed for liver cancer? When is it performed?

Liver transplantation is sometimes recommended for patients with hepatocellular carcinoma for several reasons. First, the entire liver is removed as part of liver transplantation. This removes the tumor as well as any single cells that may have spread from the tumor to other areas of the liver; these usually would not be taken care of by a regular surgical resection that eliminates only the tumors seen to the naked eye of the surgeon. These microscopic cells, if present, may result in tumor recurrence if just part of the liver is removed. In fact, in the vast majority of patients whose tumor returns, it recurs in only the remaining portion of the liver. The other major rationale to remove the entire liver exists for patients with cirrhosis. The new liver will have normal function, and thus, the patient will no longer be at risk for the complications of cirrhosis. Nevertheless, viral hepatitis infection may recur in the new liver, and continued excessive alcohol use may affect the function of the new liver.

Various guidelines exist that state which patients with liver cancer should receive a liver transplant. The most widely used in this country are as follows: a single tumor that is less than 5 cm or three tumors that are each less than 3 cm, no evidence of blood vessel invasion on radiologic studies, and no evidence of cancer that has spread outside the liver. Tumor invasion of blood vessels identifies patients who are at high risk for having the tumor spread to other areas of their body, and patients with blood vessel invasion, as well as those with tumors larger than 5 cm or many tumors, may have less benefit from a liver transplantation. Other important factors, such as patient age, exist. Patients over 70 years old are less likely to be considered candidates for transplantation. Other factors that may make you ineligible for a liver transplant are severe heart or lung disease, active alcohol abuse, prior cancer, active infection, or a psychiatric condition that may interfere with your ability to comply with medical care.

It is important to know that a proper clinical trial has never been performed to determine whether liver resection or liver transplantation is better. Such a trial would be difficult to conduct, as patients would have to consent to receiving one of the two treatments in a randomized way (e.g., by tossing a coin). Based on numerous published series of liver resection and transplantation, the survival appears similar between the two treatments, although this topic is highly controversial among doctors.

Because my father had recovered successfully from an unrelated colon cancer over a decade ago, this made him an unlikely (low priority) organ candidate. We were advised that liver transplantation was not appropriate for him. The major problems with liver transplantation, from a caregiver's point of view, are not only the long waiting period, but also deciding when to pursue a liver transplant as the first option.

47. From where do new livers come?

A new liver may come from one of two sources: A cadaver liver is obtained from a person whose brain has died but his or her organs are still alive. For instance, a person may die in an automobile accident, but his or her organs remain functional for a short period of time thereafter. The organs are donated for transplantation if the family agrees or the donor wished it so. An international organization called United Network for Organ Sharing (UNOS) distributes the available organs to patients on the transplant waiting list. Patients are given organs based on their degree of liver function and whether they have biological similarities with the donor (blood type and body size). The waiting time for a liver is variable but could be as long as a few years because there is a shortage of donor livers compared with the number of patients who need liver transplants.

UNOS prioritizes patients to receive a cadaveric liver with a scoring system. The **MELD** (model for end-stage liver disease) is a score that is based on your blood work. Specifically, your **creatinine** (which reflects kidney function), **bilirubin**, and **prothrombin** time (which reflect liver function) determine your score. The score ranges from 6 to 40. The higher your score, the more likely that you will receive a liver. Patients with cancer are given an additional number of points. Otherwise, many of them would never get an organ because there are many patients in full liver failure without cancer who would get priority.

The other source of a new liver is from a living donor. A family member or friend agrees to donate part of their liver. In many cases, this may significantly extend the patient's life and prevent the patient from dying while on a waiting list for a cadaveric liver. Every effort is made to minimize potential complications to the donor. However, liver resection is a major operation. Rarely, people have died donating a portion of their liver to someone else.

To give you an idea of how liver transplantation is used for hepatocellular cancer, 5,326 liver transplants were performed in the United States in 2002. Of them, 1,068 were performed for hepatocellular cancer, of which 37 involved a live donor.

48. How am I evaluated for a liver transplant?

Liver transplantation is carried out at specialized centers. The evaluation process is quite extensive, as liver transplantation is such a large operation and donor liv-

MELD (model for end-stage liver disease)

a mathematical equation that is used to prioritize patients for liver transplantation based on their laboratory values.

Creatinine

a substance usually excreted from the body through urine. It is used to help assess kidney function.

Bilirubin

a component of bile that comes from the breakdown of red blood cells.

Prothrombin

a protein produced by the liver that helps blood to clot.

ers are scarce. You will undergo extensive blood testing. In particular, you will be tested for previous hepatitis infection and **human immunodeficiency virus** (HIV), the virus that is responsible for AIDS. You will have several radiologic tests that may include a CT scan, an MRI, an ultrasound, an **endoscopy** to determine whether you have varices, and an **arteriography** to look at your blood vessels. The remainder of the evaluation will be like that described for liver resection.

Numerous types of doctors and associated health care personnel who work together will determine whether you are a suitable candidate for a liver transplant. These doctors include a transplant surgeon, a hepatologist, a transplant coordinator who will work with you closely before and after a transplant, and a social worker, a psychologist, or a psychiatrist who will help you and your family handle the psychologic stress of undergoing a transplant.

49. What will happen while I am on the waiting list?

If you are placed on a transplant waiting list for a cadaveric liver, you will be evaluated periodically to assess your liver function and the extent of your tumor. While you are waiting, your doctors may want to treat your cancer and may recommend a localized procedure, including a hepatic artery embolization, alcohol injection, radiofrequency ablation, or less commonly, a surgical resection.

You will be monitored regularly (e.g., every 3 months) to determine the extent of your tumor. You do run the risk of your tumor progressing to the point that you are no longer eligible for transplantation. While waiting, some patients actually die because of liver failure

Human immuno-deficiency virus (HIV)

a virus that destroys helper cells of the immune system that usually fight infections and may lead to AIDS.

Endoscopy

a procedure that allows a gastroenterologist to look at the inside of the stomach and the first part of the intestine to search for dilated blood vessels (varices), ulcers, or gastritis.

Arteriography

a radiologic test that demonstrates the artery branches of a person. Arteriography is used to identify the artery branches that supply a tumor during hepatic artery embolization.

Treatment

or tumor progression. You may no longer be eligible for a transplant if your tumor progresses because you may no longer fulfill the criteria for a transplant (see Question 46). In other words, if your tumor becomes extensive, a transplant may not help you anymore.

50. What is involved in a cadaveric liver transplant?

You will be notified immediately if a cadaver liver organ becomes available. You will be rushed into the hospital and prepared for surgery. Occasionally, the donor liver will be found to be inadequate or not suitable for you, and the intended transplant will be aborted. You will then go back on the waiting list. If the organ is suitable, you then will undergo a 4- to 8-hour operation to remove your existing liver and to implant the new liver. After the operation, you will be placed in the intensive care unit for generally a few days while you are recovering. You will have multiple tubes in your body to help your doctors take better care of you. Your blood work will be monitored very closely. You can expect to spend 1 to 2 weeks in the hospital recovering. During this time, you will be taught about the new medications that you must take to reduce your immune function so that your body does not reject your new liver.

51. What is involved in a living related liver transplantation?

If you receive a living related donor liver, you and the donor will generally be admitted the morning of surgery. The donor operation will take about 3 to 4 hours, and the donor will be in the hospital for about 5 to 7 days. You will be given part of the donor's liver. The newly transplanted part will undergo regeneration in your body to provide you with a normal-sized liver.

52. What are the complications of liver transplantation?

Because of the technical complexity of performing a liver transplant and the immunologic aspects of receiving a new liver, several potential complications exist after liver transplantation:

1. Bleeding: Just as with liver resection, occasionally a patient must undergo another operation for bleeding shortly after the original operation.

2. Hepatic artery clotting or **thrombosis**: Sometimes, the hepatic artery, which is one of the blood vessels that supplies the liver with fresh blood, can clot. Another operation may be needed to address this problem. In the worst case, another liver transplant may have to be performed.

3. Primary liver nonfunction: In some patients, the new liver fails to work properly for unexplained reasons. Another liver may have to be transplanted immediately

4. Biliary leak: In some patients, bile can leak from the connection of the old bile duct to the new bile duct. This usually resolves with conservative therapy.

5. Infection: Infection can occur at anytime after transplantation because you will be taking medication that suppresses your **immune system**. You will be

Thrombosis

the formation of clots.

Immune system

an intricate body system that protects people against foreign organisms or toxins that may cause disease.

taught that any sign of infection requires immediate medical attention because otherwise, even with a minor infection, your life could be threatened.

6. Rejection: Your body may try to reject your new liver. Generally, **rejection** can be stopped by altering the immune-suppressing drugs that you are taking. A liver biopsy performed by placing a needle in your side may be performed to diagnose the extent of the rejection. It is very important to take your medications and to comply with frequent medical monitoring to avoid rejection.

7. Recurrent hepatitis: Most patients with chronic hepatitis B or C will have recurrence of hepatitis in the new liver. The concern is that the virus is still circulating in the blood of a patient previously infected with hepatitis and can relocate and attack the new liver, thus causing hepatitis.

Rejection

the process by which the body refuses a donated transplanted liver and regards it as foreign.

53. Will I be cured after a liver transplantation?

Overall, liver transplantation is safe and highly successful. In patients without liver cancer, the 1-year survival is approximately 90%, and the 5-year survival is approximately 80%. In patients with liver cancer, survival is mostly determined by whether the tumor returns. The 5-year survival is generally between 50% and 75%. The resumption of a normal quality of life is expected.

54. Can I suppress the hepatitis from recurring and infecting the new liver?

Using interferon (see Question 10) to suppress virus replication, one might hope to reduce the damage to the liver cells and thus decrease the risk of developing cancer again. So far, the data have been controversial. Interferon itself may cause inflammation in the liver. Thus, this therapy should not be considered routine. Such therapy should preferably be given as part of a **clinical trial** and after reviewing the benefits and risks with your doctor.

55. What is tumor ablation?

Ablation is the destruction of a tumor without actually removing it. In some cases, the entire tumor can be destroyed, especially if the tumor is less than 3 cm in diameter. With larger tumors, it is more likely that a small part of the tumor will survive and begin to grow again at some point. Several techniques of ablation exist; hepatic artery embolization, alcohol injection, radiofrequency ablation, and cryotherapy are the most widely used. Each method acts in a different way, as described later. Some physicians will use them in combination. For instance, an embolization can be performed one day, followed by radiofrequency ablation or an alcohol injection the next. Any of the various procedures can be repeated in the future if your tumor grows back. If you have multiple or large tumors, your doctors may elect to apply those procedures a few times within the first 2 months of diagnosis, in order to treat all of your cancer. However, your multidisciplinary team needs to discuss this to ensure that only appropriate therapy is considered; other beneficial therapies, such as chemotherapy, are discussed as well.

56. What is hepatic artery embolization?

Hepatic artery embolization is the injection of particles into the hepatic artery in order to destroy the tumor. The particles can be thought of as microscopic

Clinical trial
a research study that answers many of the questions regarding newly discovered therapies.

Treatment

sand that clogs the blood vessels feeding the tumor. Hepatocellular carcinoma depends largely on blood supplied by the hepatic artery to survive. Part of the hepatic artery can be clogged because your liver receives blood from another vessel called the portal vein. Many doctors use particles that have a chemotherapy agent attached to them. It is unclear whether particles alone or particles with attached chemotherapy are better to use. Each group of doctors has its preference based on experience.

A special type of radiologist called an **interventional radiologist** performs hepatic artery embolization. These radiologists are specialized in performing invasive procedures under x-ray technology guidance. Usually, you come into the hospital on the day of the procedure. The procedure takes about 2 hours. You will be put to light sleep. The procedure is carried out while you are lying flat on a table. The skin in your leg (usually the right leg) is numbed with a tiny injection. Then a small tube is placed into the main artery in your leg. An x-ray machine is positioned above you and is used to monitor the location of the small tube, which is passed through a large artery called the **aorta** and then into the hepatic artery, which feeds your liver. The tube is advanced into either the right or left branch of the hepatic artery. From there, particles can be released. In general, it is more desirable to occlude selectively the specific blood vessels that are supplying a tumor and to preserve the vessels going to a normal liver. At the end of the procedure, the small tube is removed from your leg. You will have to lay flat for 4 to 6 hours afterward to make sure that the wound does not bleed and heals well.

Interventional radiologist

a doctor who specializes in performing procedures under radiologic (ultrasound, x-ray, or CT scan) guidance such as tumor biopsies and hepatic artery embolization

Aorta

the largest artery in the body. It originates from the heart, and its branches supply the entire body with blood containing oxygen.

Embolization can cause a number of side effects; thus, most patients are admitted to the hospital for 2 to 4 days. In general, the magnitude of the side effects is proportional to the amount of tumor that is destroyed. If you have a large tumor, you can expect to have a lot of side effects if it was completely embolized because of the amount of dead tissue that results from the embolization. Dead tissue releases a lot of toxic substances into your bloodstream; these toxins can make you sick. You may develop a fever. Another common side effect is **nausea**. This can be controlled with special medication, but you may not wish to eat for a day or so. Pain can occur, and you will receive pain medication for relief. Rarely, embolization will cause a problem with your heart or kidney function. Another unusual complication is the formation of an infection in the dead tumor tissue. This is called an **abscess**, and then you will be treated with **antibiotics**. In rare situations, you may need a drain placed into the infection. Also, the artery in your leg may be adversely affected by the tube that was temporarily placed there during the procedure. Bleeding can occur at the puncture site and form a large bruise called a **hematoma**. Occasionally, a patient may require an operation to repair the blood vessel if it was damaged.

Nausea

the feeling of sickness in the stomach with an urge to vomit.

Abscess

a collection of pus.

Antibiotics

medications used to fight infections.

Hematoma

a collection of blood.

57. What is radiofrequency ablation and cryotherapy?

Radiofrequency ablation and cryotherapy are used to destroy a tumor by inserting a metal probe into the tumor and exposing it to extremes of temperature. Radiofrequency ablation heats the tumor, whereas cryotherapy freezes it. Radiofrequency ablation and cryotherapy can only be used if you have a limited number of tumors (usually less than five or six) that are small to medium in size (less than 5 cm). Either procedure can be performed in a variety of ways. An interventional radiologist can place the probe percutaneously (meaning through the skin), in which case sedation will be required during the procedure. Radiofrequency ablation and cryotherapy can also be performed via laparoscopy or during an open surgical operation. In those cases, both require general anesthesia. Laparoscopy involves several small incisions in your abdomen. Open laparotomy is performed through a cut in your belly. Your doctor will decide which access you require based on the number, size, and location of your tumors. For instance, not all liver tumors can be reached via the percutaneous approach. It is important to know that not all tumors can be treated with radiofrequency ablation or cryotherapy. If a tumor is close to a main bile duct, the use of these techniques may be too risky. If a tumor is near a large blood vessel, radiofrequency ablation and cryotherapy may not be advisable.

58. What is alcohol injection?

Exposure to pure alcohol can directly kill cells. Many patients with hepatocellular carcinoma have firm or hard livers because of their cirrhosis. In contrast, the tumors are quite soft. When alcohol is injected directly into a tumor, the tumor soaks it up, whereas the surrounding firm liver does not. This is the basis for using an alcohol injection. Alcohol injection is normally performed percutaneously. Just as with radiofrequency ablation and cryotherapy, the number, size, and location of your tumors are important in determining whether alcohol injection can be performed.

The treatment is administered by an interventional radiologist, who guides a needle while the patient is under anesthesia.

My father suffered only minor local pain on his right side after each alcohol injection treatment. Sometimes the injection was accompanied by embolization. Basically, the tumor is attacked in two ways: starved of its blood supply and then dried out by the alcohol. Usually, about a day after treatment, my father would start to run a low-grade fever for a day or two. In general, he tolerated the injections very well. A month later, the CT scans would sometimes show that the center of the tumors was of a different contrast, meaning that some of the tumor cells had necrosed (died).

59. What is chemotherapy?

Chemotherapy is the use of particular chemicals to kill or arrest the growth of cancer cells. Another name that implies the same function is **cytotoxic drugs** (cyto derives from cytology, which is the study of cells). Chemotherapy agents are commonly given intravenously through a needle in the arm, although a few can be given orally as pills. Chemotherapy will thus be available throughout the body or systemically and not only at selective sites such as the liver. This carries the advantage of treating the cancer at multiple sites in case it has already spread to different sites in the liver or even outside of the liver.

Cytotoxic drugs

chemical substances that are used as chemotherapy to kill cancer cells.

How often chemotherapy is given depends on the drug or combination of drugs based on the nature of the disease and the patient's condition. Generally, chemotherapy may be given weekly to once every 3 weeks. This does not mean that more frequent delivery of drugs is more effective. A given drug may be given in a variety of ways.

Just as chemotherapy might kill dividing cancer cells, it might also harm normal cells in the body that divide rapidly, such as hair follicles, the lining of the guts, and different blood cells. This produces unwanted side effects, or toxicity. The normal cells, however, have an inherent ability to repair and replace the destroyed cells—something cancer cells commonly cannot do because they lack the necessary repair mechanisms.

Body surface area

a measurement used to dose chemotherapy based on a patient's height and weight.

To correct for the different sizes of patients, doctors use something called the **body surface area** (BSA). The dose of chemotherapy is determined based on BSA. BSA is calculated from the height and weight of a patient. You may notice that your chemotherapy dose is listed in mg/m^2. This is milligrams (amount of the drug) per square meter (this is your body surface area). This method ensures that a tall or heavy patient would not be undertreated and also that a very short or thin patient would not be overtreated.

60. What is the chemotherapy standard of care to treat advanced primary liver cancer?

The National Comprehensive Cancer Center Network does not list any chemotherapy agent as a standard of care for primary liver cancer. It does recommend, however, that patients with advanced-stage primary liver cancer join a clinical trial (see Question 61) that is evaluating a new drug or a combination of existing/new drugs. We agree with this recommendation and encourage patients to join clinical trials whenever possible. However, we recognize that this may be difficult for many reasons:

1. Clinical trials are not available in all communities throughout the country. Several are available only

at large, comprehensive cancer centers. However, patients should still ask their physicians about this option, as many trials are available to community physicians through cooperative groups.

2. Primary liver cancer is not common in the United States, even though it is one of the most common cancers in the world. A concern exists that its incidence in the United States is on the rise, especially with the increasing prevalence of hepatitis C. This fact and the global aspect of this disease may help bring more awareness and more interest in developing clinical trials.

3. Not all patients are candidates for clinical trials. Clinical trials are designed to answer specific questions within the boundaries of specific criteria that a certain patient might or might not have. This does not imply that patients who are not eligible for a clinical trial should not be treated with any therapy. Thus, other treatments outside of a clinical trial can be recommended.

61. What is a clinical trial?

A clinical trial is a research study that answers many of the questions regarding newly discovered therapies. Medical researchers discover new therapies daily and describe their mode of action with an evolving precision. Over decades, newly discovered therapies must be tested in patients to establish their safety and efficacy.

Clinical trials can answer many scientific and medical questions, which range from testing new drugs, a combination of known drugs, and the method of administering certain drugs or testing new therapies such as radiation, studying nutrition, and behavior. The basic rules, which are discussed later, generally apply to all clinical trials; however, we discuss them in the context of hepatocellular carcinoma.

All clinical trials are, and always should be, detailed and clearly described in a manuscript called a **protocol**. A protocol is the ultimate reference for clinical trials. It describes all of the rules and conditions that govern the trial. This ensures the quality of the trial and thus its reproducibility, as well as the safety and protection of the patients on the trial.

Unfortunately, history tells us about badly conducted clinical trials that might have exploited patients for the sake of answering a scientific question. However, nowadays, patients should not fear joining a clinical trial when clinically indicated, as all protocols are now governed by federal regulations that protect all patients. These rules and many other ethical considerations are monitored very closely by an **institutional review board**. Patients who are given the option to join a clinical trial make the ultimate decision about whether to participate. If the patient does enter a trial, he or she has the right to withdraw from the trial at any time. These rights, as well the details of the study, should be discussed between the patient and the physician in a process called the informed consent, which culminates in both signing an agreement that includes all of the details discussed. This ensures the coherence of the study and protects the rights of all patients.

Clinical trials generally happen in three phases: phase I, II, and III. The goal of a phase I study is primarily to establish the safety of a newly discovered drug or

Protocol

a detailed description of all of the rules and conditions that govern a clinical trial. A protocol is the ultimate reference for a clinical trial.

Institutional review board

a collective board that oversees all clinical trials. The board generally includes doctors, researchers, lawyers, administrators, pharmacists, and patients' advocates.

combination of drugs while studying the efficacy in many diseases. A phase II trial studies primarily the efficacy of a drug or a combination of drugs in a specific disease. However, the ultimate answer on efficacy is usually sought through a phase III study that compares the experimental drug or drugs to the standard care of this disease. In a phase III trial, patients will be randomly assigned to either arms of the study (experimental versus standard) to ensure the validity of the experiment, and may be blinded to the assigned arm.

During the last year of my father's treatment, we explored further options with the doctors, including new chemotherapy drug trials. Unfortunately, by this point, his deteriorating liver condition (multiple tumors, ascites, and low blood protein levels) precluded him from qualifying for many of the trials. Still, that did not prevent me from doing research on the Internet to find out what new phase II and III trials were being offered and whether my father was eligible. I would fax short descriptions of the drug trials to my father's nurse at the clinic and ask her to follow up with doctors before his next scheduled visit. This kept me actively involved in my father's care and offered us hope.

62. Where can I find out about clinical trials for liver cancer, and how do I know which trial is best for me?

Patients should ask their doctors about clinical trials. Many doctors both at academic centers and in private practices in the community run or are part of a group of doctors running a clinical trial. Thus, the answer might be at the doorstep of where a patient lives. Nonetheless, patients might consider commuting a reasonable distance to get to a center that runs a pertinent clinical trial. Patients might know about those through either their doctors, medical centers' websites, or the government National Cancer Institute websites: *www.cancer.gov* and *www.clinicaltrials.gov*. The National Cancer Institute offers not only a listing of all clinical trials that are registered with them, but also several web pages with information about clinical trials. Other sites that offer similar services include the Coalition of National Cancer Cooperative Groups, *www.cancertrialshelp.org*, and Centerwatch, *www.centerwatch.com*.

If a patient identifies a clinical trial that is relevant to his or her medical condition, he or she should discuss the trial further with his or her doctor. The doctor might call the investigators and find out more about the trial. This can ensure that patients will seek only trials that they might be eligible for and save a lot of frustration and travel time and expenses. If a patient is deemed ineligible for a certain trial, he or she should not be disappointed or have feelings of hopelessness. It is important that certain clinical trials answer only a specific question in a specific subset of patients with a given disease. For example, a new drug for primary liver cancer may be only tested in patients who have a specific level of liver function, and this does not reflect on your illness level if you are not eligible.

63. What chemotherapy drugs might be used to treat liver cancer outside of a clinical trial?

Doxorubicin (Adriamycin) remains the most studied chemotherapy in primary liver cancer. Doxorubicin was never established as a standard of care for this disease because of varied response rates that were difficult to interpret. Recently, however, a phase III clinical trial used doxorubicin as single therapy in its standard arm. Thus, it is a valid option that should be offered to patients. Undoubtedly, with the pace at which new data on other single-agent or combination therapies are being published, our recommendation might change soon. In all instances, it is very important for patients and their physicians to discuss the different options that are available. Doxorubicin is infused intravenously through the arm. Extreme vigilance, however, is necessary because if the IV malfunctions, the drug might seep into the skin and cause permanent damage. Usually, the nurses infusing the drug are highly trained and qualified to avoid this problem. Nonetheless, as the drug is being infused, patients should warn the nurses immediately if they witness any pain, discoloration, or burning at the infusion site.

64. Is receiving more than one chemotherapy drug better?

Many attempts have been made to improve on the efficacy of single-agent doxorubicin by adding other drugs. Other drug combinations without doxorubicin have also been tested. The only combination that has been tested in a phase III trial against single-agent doxorubicin is doxorubicin plus cisplatin, 5-fluorouracil, and interferon—a combination that is known as PIAF. Overall, the results do not support the routine use of PIAF. However, a careful interpretation of these data and data from a phase II study of the same combination justifies using PIAF in some patients who might benefit from chemotherapy in an aim to shrink their tumor and render it resectable by surgery. Such a strategy should be considered carefully where applicable, and any decision should involve your medical oncologist and surgeon.

65. How will I know that the chemotherapy treatment is working?

Radiologic imaging and AFP evaluations are the two objective ways of assessing response to chemotherapy in liver cancer. They are complementary; however, one must be careful not to use AFP alone as the only indicator of response.

Doctors routinely will use a CT scan, an MRI, or an ultrasound as a baseline before starting any treatment. As many patients who receive chemotherapy have metastatic disease (stage IV), a CT scan or an MRI of the whole body would be the most reasonable modality to use. You can expect to have a repeat evaluation, preferably using the same radiologic technique every 2 to 3 months. Any CT scan studying the liver itself should be done using a technique called **triphasic CT**. Primary liver cancer lesions are notorious for being difficult to see on CT scan; however, taking pictures during three different phases of the blood flow through the liver makes the interpretation of such CT a scan much easier.

Triphasic CT
a CT scan that evaluates the liver at three phases of the blood flow through it.

Stage IV, or metastatic disease, is treatable but is almost always incurable. Therapy becomes part of patient's life. Any benefit other than shrinking or stabilizing the tumor, such as improvement in pain control and performance and increased appetite (called clinical benefit response), has not been studied in primary liver cancer, but anecdotally, many patients notice that they felt better or have an improved level of function while they were receiving chemotherapy. Patients should thus lead their lives normally, and the outcome of the therapy should be assessed personally on a daily basis and clinically on a regular basis. CT scans and MRI results should be no more than a benchmark to assure both patients and physicians that they are on the right track; they should never be the goal itself. Patients would appreciate this approach very much as they see themselves going back in the flow of life as able as they can and do not live just until the next scan.

66. How is the response to therapy assessed on a CT scan or an MRI?

Radiologic evaluations are generally descriptive. The radiologist can evaluate the cancer in the liver and elsewhere and measure it generally in two dimensions and possibly three. Those measurements are compared with a baseline CT scan or an MRI before the start of therapy and with scans obtained later while on therapy.

The best result would be a complete response to therapy, where the cancer would disappear completely on the radiologic studies performed. This is an extremely rare phenomenon in primary liver cancer.

A partial response means a reduction in the volume of cancer by 50% or more. In the case of doxorubicin, the chance of that happening is 12%. In that instance, the recommendation would be to continue on the same treatment if the patient is feeling well and if the liver function allows it.

Stable disease implies that the tumor did not grow in size or that it grew less than 25%. This 25% margin of error allows correcting for technical variations of the radiologic studies. Stable disease is an acceptable reason for continuing the same treatment. Although it is preferable that the cancer shrinks or decreases in size, preventing it from growing is also beneficial. In this case, the same treatment is generally continued.

An increase in tumor size of more than 25% represents "progression of disease." This is a reason to stop the current treatment and to consider an alternative.

67. What are some of the general side effects of chemotherapy?

General side effects can be expected with any chemotherapy treatment, but others are specific to a certain drug or combination of drugs. Because chemotherapy kills reproducing cancer cells, it can be expected that it can kill normal reproducing cells. However, because these normal cells are genetically healthy, they can reproduce again.

Red blood cells

cells that carry oxygen and carbon dioxide. They are red because of their high load of iron, which is essential to their function.

White blood cells

cells that help fight infection.

Platelets

pieces of cells that float in the blood and promote clotting where necessary.

An expected general side effect of chemotherapy is the destruction of **red blood cells** that carry oxygen, **white blood cells** that fight infections, and **platelets** that are responsible for clotting blood. The caring oncologist should monitor these carefully through routine blood work. Patients will be warned at the same time to mention extra signs of fatigue, which is partly explained by a lower number of red cells. Physicians might give weekly skin injections of erythropoietin (Procrit®) or every other week darbepoetin alfa (Aranesp®), which help the body produce more red cells. Not all fatigue symptoms are due to low red blood cells. Patients with primary liver cancer might be tired because of their illness, and the chemotherapy itself might undoubtedly cause tiredness. Infections are possible because of the possible reduced number of white cells. Any sign of fever should prompt a call to the physician and even a possible visit to the hospital. A physician again might elect to give a certain skin injection to boost the number of white cells (Neupogen®, Neulasta®, Filgrastim®). This is not necessarily done even if the white count is low, as it depends on the chemotherapy scheduling and some other factors. Bleeding through the mouth, rectum, or other sites is of critical importance, especially in primary liver cancer, where the number of platelets could be low to start with due to liver failure or cirrhosis (see Question 88). Physicians might elect to give chemotherapy for patients with platelet levels that are lower than the commonly used reference of 100,000 per mcL; however, this requires extreme vigilance by both the patient and physician. It is difficult to justify giving any chemotherapy below a platlet count of 75,000 per mcL.

Most chemotherapy agents cause nausea and possibly vomiting, but to variable extents. Because these symptoms are predictable, patients most likely will be taught about the potential nausea and will be given supportive medications to prevent it or alleviate it. One form of nausea is anticipatory that a patient might have learned because of poor control of nausea and/or vomiting with previous chemotherapy treatments. This stresses the importance of controlling nausea as tightly as possible. The good thing is that there are now many drugs to help with even severe nausea.

Most importantly, it is very difficult to know or tell how you may react to chemotherapy. Patients may have none of those side effects, all of them, or some of them. In anticipation, it is good to learn about all that might happen and inform your doctor of any symptoms that seems unusual or unexpected. When the oncologist informs you about all potential side effects, you should not be discouraged or consider not being treated.

68. What are some side effects of Doxorubicin (Adriamycin)?

In addition, doxorubicin may cause diarrhea and mouth sores. However, these two effects are generally tolerable and would not cause any limitation on administering the chemotherapy. Patients may also notice a discoloration of their urine, which might appear darker. Darkening of the nails may also occur. Rarely, patients may develop a skin rash or an allergic reaction. Patients will often lose their hair, but it will regrow within 3 months after stopping the medication.

Doxorubicin might also affect heart function. This may occur acutely within the first 2 to 3 days of starting treatment. Patients may feel a skip or rapid heart beats or positional pain in their chest. These usually are self-limiting and dissipate rapidly. Nevertheless, a doctor should be informed of any such symptoms. On the other hand, as patients receive increasing amounts of doxorubicin, the drug may accumulate to a toxic level in their heart. This might affect the heart function. Doctors should monitor the heart function of the patient very closely. Patients should have a MUGA scan (**MUltiple Gated Acquisition scan**) at baseline and routinely after a few cycles of treatment. The MUGA is a noninvasive test that produces a moving image of the heart. From this image, the health of the heart's major pumping chamber (the left ventricle) can be assessed. The frequency at which the MUGA scans will be obtained will decrease as a patient continues to

Multiple gated acquisition scan (MUGA)

a noninvasive test that produces a moving image of the heart and assesses function level.

receive more doxorubicin. Even if the heart is functioning well, doctors may advise against continuing administering doxorubicin beyond a cumulative dose of 550 mg/m^2. Beyond this dose, patients are at risk of developing heart failure. This is equivalent to about 9 to 10 doses of therapy (at 60 mg/m^2).

69. What are biologic and targeted therapies?

Nowadays, scientists have come to a better understanding of how cancer cells keep producing. We now know of specific steps during cell reproduction that lead to this uncontrolled replication of cells, which causes cancer. We have also identified specific therapies that stop tumor replication or disrupt its blood supply. Like for many other cancers, these new "targeted" or "biologic" therapies might play a role in primary liver cancer. Many of them are being tested in different clinical trials, but as of the time that this book is published, none was approved for the treatment of primary liver cancer. Although we call them targeted therapies, they are not as specific as one might think, and thus, they can have side effects the same way chemotherapy does. Pending their approval, we strongly recommend against their use outside of a clinical trial, as their safety profile is not fully understood, especially in liver cancer. As discussed before, the complexity of the disease and the liver failure or cirrhosis that might be present could cause more challenges on to how to deliver these new drugs. Thus drugs, such as bevacizumab (Avastin®), gefitinib (Iressa®), or cetuximab (Erbitux®), should not be used outside of a clinical trial until further evaluations and approval are completed.

70. What is liver pump chemotherapy?

Some patients might have cancer in only the liver that is, however, scattered throughout the liver. This situation, as explained before, may not be amenable to surgery, transplant, or any other of the local therapies previously discussed. However, chemotherapy might be given only where needed in the liver, thus maximizing its effectiveness against the disease and minimizing any possible systemic side effects. This therapy entails having a simple catheter inserted into an artery that leads to your liver, through which chemotherapy is given. Another possibility is having a **pump** placed under the skin in the wall of your abdomen; it is connected to an artery that leads to the liver. The pump can be accessed through the skin like a **mediport** (Question 82). The drug that is administered through the pump will be delivered to your liver, however, over a longer period of time, generally 2 weeks, thus exposing the tumor to more chemotherapy. Many studies have been done about this form of therapy; however, until now, at least in the United Stated, this is not considered a standard of care. This is offered at many cancer centers as part of ongoing clinical trials.

Pump

a pump system used to deliver chemotherapy at a fixed rate and for a specific period of time.

Mediport

a half-dollar sized, round well that is connected to a tube that is used for the delivery of medication within a vein. The entire apparatus sits underneath the skin and is inserted during a small procedure.

71. What happens during a chemotherapy session?

Most, if not all, chemotherapy is now given in the outpatient setting. It is rare that you need to be admitted to the hospital to receive chemotherapy. On the day of treatment, you might or might not need to see your medical oncologist—depending on where you stand in your treatment and how well you are doing. You will have your blood work checked first. This is critically important, as many of the chemotherapy drugs affect your white and red blood cells and platelets (see Question 67). If your blood work shows those cell levels to be in the safe range, then you will proceed to chemotherapy. You will sit in a comfortable chair (like a lazy chair), and an IV will be attached to your arm or mediport, if you have one (see Question 82). You will be given a series of some medications, mainly to prevent acute side effects such as nausea, vomiting, diarrhea, or allergic reactions, depending on which drug you are receiving and your previous experience with the drug. Then chemotherapy will be administered. This might take a few minutes to a few hours depending on which drug is being infused. Some of them may need to be given slowly. The experience is comfortable. There should be no pain involved. However, if you feel any burning in your arm, you need to tell the nurse immediately, as the IV might have leaked some of the chemotherapy under the skin (see Question 63). You can watch TV, read a magazine, or read this book and then have breakfast or lunch after any nausea is under control. At the completion of the chemotherapy, you may need further fluid hydration. At the end of the session, you are disconnected and can go home. You should not drive yourself, as you most likely received some antinausea medicines that could cause drowsiness. Check with your doctor.

72. What happens in the few days after I receive chemotherapy?

Side effects will vary depending on which chemotherapy drugs you have received. In general, you will feel tired for a few days after the day chemotherapy is given. You might feel lazy, not up to doing things; however, after a few days, things improve, and you will regain your previous level of energy and activity. You might also have for the same period of time more nausea and possibly vomiting. This delayed nausea can last for a few days. Your doctor should already have prescribed several medications to combat nausea. You should take those medications any time that you feel nauseous. You might feel overwhelmed and fearful that any of the side effects from the drugs might happen. Use common sense in interpreting any signs or symptoms, and more importantly, do not hesitate to call your doctor to discuss any of those signs and symptoms. Your doctor might help to reassure you or might identify something more of concern that requires medical attention, another prescription, or possibly a visit to the hospital for further evaluation.

73. What is radiation therapy?

Radiation therapy
treatment against cancer that uses radiation as a form of energy to kill cancer cells.

External beam radiation
radiation therapy that is aimed at a specific site in the body and delivered from outside of the body through the skin.

Brachytherapy
radiation therapy that is applied within the body cavity.

Radiation therapy depends on the high energy of certain electromagnetic waves. These powerful radiation rays can be controlled and directed toward a cancer. The aim is obviously to kill cancer cells. The two main types of radiation waves are x-rays and gamma-rays. They differ in production and power and may have different applicability in cancer treatment. Radiation can be delivered from outside of the body, penetrate through the skin, and be targeted to where the tumor is. This is called **external beam radiation**; it usually consists of x-rays. Another form of radiation that produces gamma-rays from radioactive material can be inserted or implanted inside the body next to where the tumor is. This is called **brachytherapy**.

74. Can radiation be used to treat liver cancer?

Although radiation is a commonly used form of treatment for many cancers, its role in the case of primary liver cancer is rather limited because the liver has poor tolerance to radiation. Generally, the number of treatments to the liver will not be more than 10. These are usually delivered daily Monday to Friday over 1 week. Radiating the entire liver might cause liver inflammation, called **radiation hepatitis**. This problem can be overcome by using localized radiation therapy to where it is needed in the liver. Doctors who treat cancer patients with radiation (also called radiation oncologists) can prepare a three-dimensional computer model of your liver and the tumor and then target a small radiation therapy emitted from many sources to a very localized focus of tumor where the effect of the sum of all those small amounts of radiation will maximize and cause tumor damage without affecting the surrounding liver tissue. Because of the limitations of radiation in liver cancer, the role of radiation therapy in hepatocellular carcinoma may be limited to palliation and control of pain if any.

Radiation hepatitis inflammatory damage to the liver that may be caused by radiation therapy.

75. What are Yttrium-90 microspheres?

New advances in radiation have expanded its use in hepatocellular carcinoma. Highly potent radioactive material can be attached to glass beads that can be infused into the hepatic artery and lodge next to and into tumors that are regularly fed by the hepatic artery. **Yttrium-90 microspheres**, also known as Theraspheres, have been studied in the liver since the late 1980s and have been proven to be active in multiple

Yttrium-90 microspheres small beads tagged with radioactive Yttrium that are delivered into the liver and lodge inside the small arteries to deliver their anti-cancer therapeutic effect.

clinical trials. However, so far, no studies have compared the efficacy or safety of Yttrium-90 microspheres to systemic chemotherapy.

76. What are the side effects of radiation?

The side effects of radiation therapy depend on the part of the body that is being irradiated. After radiating the liver, the overlying skin will be the first to be damaged by the radiation. You may notice it to be darker and dry, both over the abdomen and the back. Rarely, the skin might burn and appear red. The liver itself, as mentioned already, may sustain further damage secondary to radiation. This will be critical, especially if it is already cirrhotic. The closeness to the stomach might cause nausea, vomiting, and irritation of the lining of the stomach. You may also have diarrhea, as the radiation might also affect the lining of the bowels, which are in close proximity to the field of radiation. Radiation also generally causes fatigue. Finally, patients might have reduced white cells, red cells, or platelets, as the radiation might injure their production site in the **bone marrow** in the vertebral column lying right behind the liver.

77. What are complementary and alternative treatments?

Complementary medicine and **alternative medicine** are acknowledged by the National Institutes of Health and the health system as another approach to therapy that would help integrate such unconventional treatments with more conventional therapies. Many cancer centers around the country now have an integrative medicine department or a section that offers alternative therapies to patients. These include, but are not limited

Bone marrow

substance that fills the bone inner cavities and is the source of red blood cells, white blood cells, and platelets.

Complementary medicine (same as alternative medicine)

medical practices (e.g., herbal medicine) that do not follow Western medicine guidelines and that may lack a scientific proof for their effectiveness.

Alternative medicine

medical practices (e.g., herbal medicine) that do not follow Western medicine guidelines and may lack scientific proof for their effectiveness.

to, alternative systems of medical practice such as **acupuncture**, **homeopathy**, and **naturopathy**. Diet and nutrition are other components. For the mind and body, many places offer psychotherapy, meditation, hypnosis, biofeedback, and massage, among many others. You may also seek herbal remedies and other medicines that are still considered alternative by nature as they lack a clear indication by Western medicine standards.

A lot of research has undoubtedly proven some of these therapies to be effective. Discuss your interest in these methods with your doctor, who might refer you to an integrative medicine doctor. Avoid taking any medicines on your own unless you discuss it with your doctor. Remember that many medicines today are of natural origins. By the same token, many of the medicines that are labeled as natural or herbal can have potential effects and even side effects. More importantly, your doctor might help you identify the therapies that you should avoid. Oncologists nowadays know more about alternative therapies and can expect their patients to use them. Do not hesitate to discuss alternative therapies with your doctors. Bring the pills and herbs with you, and always try to have a list of ingredients. This might help your doctor identify any potentially beneficial or harmful products.

After 3 years of relatively stable health, my father's condition worsened in the fall of 2003. He had to be rushed to the hospital because of an infection. It was around then that his CT scans showed tumor growth in one of his adrenal glands. The chemotherapy regimen did not seem to be working. At that point, my family and I started to seek alternative treatments because his conventional options seemed to be running out.

Treatment

Acupuncture
a Chinese medical procedure in which fine needles are placed through the skin to relieve pain or for other treatment reasons.

Homeopathy
treating disease with small amounts of treatments that in large amounts in healthy people may produce symptoms of the same disease.

Naturopathy
the science that uses herbs and herb products as a form of therapy against disease.

Many websites and family friends touted the antitumor properties of mushrooms. Although the anecdotal evidence was very encouraging, the clinical studies, mostly in Japanese and Chinese journals, supporting these treatments are very limited at best. The theories propose that the mushrooms contain certain polysaccharides that strengthen the immune system's fight against cancer. I would advise everyone to be careful about the optimistic claims, as most are being promoted by the supplement manufacturers themselves.

After consulting with his doctors, we did give my father various mushroom extracts, along with milk thistle, an herb that is supposed to improve liver function. We figured their potential negative side-effects were small. We also tried a very risky liquid cesium treatment but stopped it after 2 weeks when my father's digestive system did not tolerate it very well. It is unknown whether these alternative treatments were beneficial to his medical condition.

78. What if my doctor recommends that no treatment should be performed?

Some patients are not eligible for any of the previously discussed treatments. Your doctor may decide that it is too risky to treat you if your tumor is too advanced, if your liver is too weak because of advanced stage cirrhosis, or if you have other significant medical problems. In this situation, your doctor will offer supportive care. This means that he or she will try to help with any symptoms that you may develop and try to maximize your quality of life. In particular, he or she will help you try to avoid further liver failure or complications from cirrhosis. This is done by helping you avoid gaining extra fluid weight by using diuretics (water pills). Other symptoms that may require treatment include mental confusion and bleeding from your stomach. You may not necessarily experience any pain, but if you do, pain medications can and should be prescribed. Some patients may also require assistance with living at home, and your physician should help arrange for a health care professional to visit you.

I believe that doctors correctly wanted to avoid doing harm to my father; thus, they stopped his treatments when they did not look like they were doing him any good. The liver is a complex chemical factory, and during cancer treatment, it is in a precarious balance. My family and I eventually came to realize that our doctors were more focused on sustaining his quality of life rather than grasping at dangerous straws for a cure.

79. How should I use the Internet to learn about my cancer?

The Internet has a vast resource of medical information. You may learn about a specialty center near you or discover a clinical trial in which you can participate. Although we recommend that you learn about your cancer, we must caution you that many times a patient will find information that is not relevant to their particular situation. This may lead to further confusion or fear. Thus, although it is valuable for you and your family to learn about hepatocellular cancer, you should discuss your research with your doctor. The value of a certain website will depend on some aspects, including the accuracy of the information. Remember that some sites are more reputable than others. Look at who is behind the website and find out whether there is any supporting staff you can contact for any questions. Make sure though that your confidentiality as a patient is kept while navigating any such sources on the Internet. The Internet may also enable you to communicate with other patients that have your disease, which may help you cope with the problems that you are facing. However, you must also be cautious about those chat rooms, as many are not monitored, and any data or information you might read needs to be placed in context.

PART SEVEN

Cancer-Related Practical Issues

I feel overwhelmed by all of the information that I am receiving. How do I make any decisions regarding my treatment?

More ...

80. I feel overwhelmed by all of the information that I am receiving. How do I make any decisions regarding my treatment?

This sentiment is understandable and expected after you have read the previous sections of this book and realized that there are many different approaches to therapy. That's good in a way, as to know that many resources are available to help. The best way to incorporate this information is to keep track of it. Take notes, but avoid immersing yourself in details because you might lose the big picture this way. In many cancer centers, you might be followed by many physicians. Your doctors will be talking to each other. It is a good idea, however, to identify one physician as the primary one, like your surgeon in case your primary therapy is a surgery or your medical oncologist if you are receiving chemotherapy.

I felt that one of the most exasperating experiences of my father's cancer was figuring out who was in charge. Because liver cancer currently has no single default method of care, but instead many avenues of treatment, during each trip to the clinic, we would have to talk to the surgeon about surgery options, the interventional radiologist about the embolization treatment options, the oncologist about chemotherapy options, the hepatobiliary specialist about hepatitis options, etc., and then we would try to assimilate all of the information ourselves. In retrospect, we maybe should have tried harder to identify a primary physician early on for my father—someone among the specialists involved who is fairly well-versed in the disease and could coordinate care among all of the other caring physicians.

81. Will changing my diet alter my cancer?

This is a common question among patients with cancer. In general, no specific diet recommendations are available for cancer patients. We would encourage you to eat a balanced diet. Your doctor may advise taking one multivitamin pill a day but most likely will advise against an intense vitamin and herbal therapy, especially if your liver is already jeopardized by the cancer itself and possibly cirrhosis if you have it. You should minimize or eliminate alcohol use. If you have cirrhosis, your doctor may limit the amount of fluid that you drink or the salt and protein that you eat. Your doctor may recommend that you seek advice from a hepatologist or a nutritionist.

As my father's cancer progressed, it became more and more difficult for him to do simple things such as swallowing foods and pills. His sense of taste was also changing. Nearly all foods lacked flavor, and he would crave a lot of salt or spice, which we tried to avoid.

In response, we would try to prepare a few foods that he liked as a special treat, such as pizza, while still encouraging him to eat the bland, healthy foods that he did not like, such as vegetables and beans. Because he had difficulty swallowing pills, we found liquid multivitamins to supplement his diet.

82. What is a mediport?

A mediport is a device that can be used to deliver chemotherapy. It may be necessary if the patient has limited intravenous access in the arms or if the chemotherapy is to be delivered continuously while the patient is at home. A mediport is inserted underneath the skin of your chest wall by a surgeon or an interventional radiologist. The procedure takes about 45 minutes and is performed while you are lightly sedated.

A mediport has two components: a reservoir and a tube. Both are underneath your skin. The reservoir is about the width of a half dollar. It may be visible as a small lump just below your collarbone. A nurse inserts a needle through your skin into the reservoir. The drug, or any other intravenous solution, then passes into a small tube that sits inside a large vein in your body.

Three main complications of having a mediport may occur. The first is that during the insertion of the device, there is an approximate 1% chance of having one of your lungs collapse. This is treated by placing a small tube into the chest and removing some air. The more common complications include infection and a blood clot. Because a mediport is a foreign object in your body, it might become infected. It is thus critical that there is an indication for a mediport and that it is not just inserted for convenience. Also, only an experienced person should access the mediport, and it should be done in a sterile fashion. Because the catheter attached to the reservoir sits in a vein, this vein may develop a clot. Your doctor may request that you take a very small dose of a blood thinner called coumadin while you have a mediport. In the case of an infection or a blood clot that is difficult to treat, your mediport may need to be removed.

83. My eyes and/or skin are yellow.

Jaundice is caused by the accumulation of bile in the body (see Question 22). It is a complication of liver failure and cirrhosis. The liver cells may be destroyed and release an overwhelming amount of bile that your body cannot absorb like it usually does and thus cause you to look yellow. By itself, jaundice is not dangerous, and at worst, it may cause itching that can be treated with an antihistamine like Benadryl® (diphenhydramine). However, the presence of jaundice, which is not as common in primary liver cancer, is a sign of a failing liver, and it could prevent you from having surgery or receiving chemotherapy, as this may further worsen your liver condition. It is not safe to give many chemotherapy drugs if the bilirubin (bile level) is elevated. Another cause of jaundice is a mechanical block in the liver that is caused by the tumor. The tumor may press on a bile duct and not allow the bile to drain the normal way to your gallbladder and intestine; thus, it backs up in the liver and blood and causes jaundice. In this case, your doctors may recommend a diverting procedure for the bile in order to decrease it and be able to treat you with chemotherapy or to relieve you of symptoms like severe itching if any.

84. How can a mechanical blockage of bile be fixed?

There are several ways to fix a blocked bile duct. One is to have a plastic or metal stent placed into your bile duct during an endoscopy. A gastroenterologist performs an endoscopy while you are lightly sedated. A scope is advanced through your mouth into your intestine. The stent is fed through the bile duct opening in your intestine. The other main way to fix a bile duct blockage is by placing a plastic tube (called a catheter) directly through your abdominal wall into the liver and then through the bile duct. Initially, bile will drain into a bag that you may place at a lower point of its insertion site under your clothes, around your waist, or around your leg. The procedure is preformed by a team of interventional radiologists while you are lightly sedated. For this, you may be admitted to the hospital and observed for few days. It may take several days for your bilirubin level to drop low enough for you to start chemotherapy again. One of the risks of the procedure is infection, and thus, you may need to be treated with antibiotics intravenously. Other complications include bleeding. This is of special concern in patients with advanced cirrhosis, as they may not clot their blood normally. This by itself may even prevent you from having the procedure. In many instances, the interventional radiologist may soon be able to place the stent permanently on the inside so that you do not have to have a bag.

85. I feel tired. Can I do anything about it?

Fatigue is a common symptom for patients with cancer. This is due to many factors. The cancer itself, especially in its advanced stages, might tire people. In addition, chemotherapy might cause fatigue, which might last for a few days after treatment. Some chemotherapy might cause a drop in the number of your red blood cells, which can also contribute to fatigue. This might be corrected by weekly skin injections of erythropoietin (Procrit®) or every other week delivery of darbepoetin alfa (Aranesp®), both of which help the body produce more red cells. This might not relieve all of the fatigue but might make you feel better.

Mental fatigue is another symptom. It results from all of the doctor appointments, tests, and the concerns and fears of having cancer. Mental fatigue is best circumvented by focusing on the daily goals and keeping notes of events so that you do not burden yourself with all of the information that you are getting. Keep it simple though, and always look at the big picture. Many relatives, friends, and colleagues will be calling to check on you. It is very good to have people around, and your doctors will always encourage you to maintain your social support group. It is also okay not to think about your cancer all of the time. You need to energize and be ready for the next step all the time.

Pain is another cause of fatigue. You have to make sure it is well controlled, as is discussed in Question 86.

I discovered simple activities that helped to revive my dad's energy and spirits. We would take short walks around the house, making it a game of how many times he could circle the kitchen before getting too tired. We rented DVDs of his favorite movies. We played board games and cards. These seemed to help take his mind off his fatigue. Even so, he took naps more frequently and did complain of sore tired muscles, particularly the upper arms, shoulders, and legs.

86. I have pain. How can I be pain free?

Pain needs to be controlled, as it might affect your mood and your function and cause you to be more ill, tired, and fatigued. You have to tell your doctor about pain because it can be alleviated. Mild pains usually respond to acetaminophen (Tylenol®) or **nonsteroidal anti-inflammatory drugs** (NSAIDs) such as Motrin® and Advil®. Acetaminophen (Tylenol®) should, however, be taken gingerly because it might affect liver function, especially in the case of advanced cirrhosis. Make sure that you tell your doctor how many Tylenol® you need and have him or her assess its safety. The NSAIDs might cause stomach bleeding, which is more possible because of the cirrhosis (see Question 90). These medications may not be enough to control your pain.

Nonsteroidal anti-inflammatory drugs

a form of medication that controls pain and inflammation that is not part of the steroid family.

In case of more severe pain, you may be prescribed opiate- or morphine-based medications. Many formulations of those medications exist; they are divided into two main categories: short-acting and long-acting. If you may require only a few pills every day, or every few days, to control your pain, your doctor will most likely prescribe a short-acting morphine such as oxycodone, one to two pills every 4 to 6 hours. These will control your pain for that period of time. Some of the short-acting opiates are a combination of Tylenol® plus oxycodone, such as Percocet®. Your doctor may avoid prescribing those for the same concerns raised with the Tylenol®, that is, liver function. If you require many short-acting pills to control pain, your doctor may elect to add a long-acting opiate that can be in the form of pills like Oxycontin®, or MS Contin®, that you take twice a day, or as a skin patch (Fentanyl®) that you apply every 3 days. Although the patch appears to be easier, you may still be prescribed pills because of allergic concerns, personal preference, or sometimes poor absorption because of reduced body fat.

Tolerance

the body's need for an increased dose of a certain medication to obtain the same effect.

The aim is to be pain free. You have to bear in mind that your pain medications requirements may increase with time because of a totally natural phenomenon called **tolerance** (this should not be confused with addiction); also, your pain may simply get worse, and you need more medications to control it. Some patients with liver cirrhosis and liver cancer, who may have acquired hepatitis through shared needles using drugs, may feel uncomfortable using opiates. You are highly encouraged to speak your fears and concerns, as assistance from your medical oncologist or even pain specialist should be available.

Like all medications, opiates have side effects. You may feel sleepy or drowsy, especially at first. This may dissipate after few days. If it persists, your medications may need to be fine tuned to reach a comfortable pain-control level, with acceptable side effects. In all instances, however, you should not operate any machinery or drive while taking opiates. Constipation is another side effect. Your bowels may become a bit sluggish while on opiates, and most likely you will need to be maintained on a daily bowel regimen of a stool softener such as Colace® and a laxative such as Senekot®, Miralax®, Magnesium citrate®, or Lactu-lose®. Drinking fluids will also help to keep you regular. You may have more or less side effects with different formulations of opiates. Sometimes switching to different medications may help to ease some of the side effects.

Cancer-Related Practical Issues

PART EIGHT

Cirrhosis–Related Practical Issues

My legs and/or my abdomen are swollen.
What can I do about it?

What is meant when my platelets are low?

More . . .

87. My legs and/or my abdomen are swollen. What can I do about it?

In the event of cirrhosis, blood pressure might build up inside the liver, causing what is called portal hypertension. This causes the body to start accumulating more water and salt, which ultimately leads to swelling in the abdomen (ascites) or in the legs (peripheral edema). The reduced ability of the cirrhotic liver to produce protein, in addition to poor nutrition, which is usually associated with cirrhosis and/or primary liver cancer, may also contribute to the swelling. When the blood vessels have a reduced amount of protein in them, they can not retain water as well. Thus, water will seep out of the blood vessels and cause **ascites** and **edema**.

As you can imagine, resolution of the fluid is unlikely to happen unless the cirrhosis improves, which may not be possible. Your doctor might still be able to help reduce the amount of accumulating fluid. The simplest way would be to restrict salt intake, as salt draws water with it. You might need to restrict your salt intake to less than 2 grams of salt (800 mg of sodium) per day. As an example, 1 slice of bread has about 500 mg of salt. Your doctor may also prescribe a water pill (diuretic) such as spironolactone (Aldactone®) or a combination of diuretics by adding furosemide (Lasix®). Usually such interventions would be sufficient at least to keep the fluid retention at a steady level. However, sometimes your doctor may also need to remove the fluid or ascites from your abdomen by inserting a needle through the skin. This is a simple bed-side procedure that could be done with or without the help of an ultrasound to localize the fluid. During the procedure, you lie on your back, probably turning more toward your right. Your doctor will

Ascites

an abnormal accumulation of fluid in the abdomen.

Edema

an abnormal accumulation of fluid in the extremities.

sterilize one spot of your skin, usually in the left lower corner of your abdomen. You will then receive numbing medicine through your skin via a needle. Afterward, your doctor will insert a needle with a catheter that will drain the clear yellowish fluid into a bottle or a bag. Your doctor will judge how much fluid should be removed to make sure that your blood pressure and heart rate are not affected by this rapid change of body fluid. The procedure carries a small risk of infection or bleeding (see Question 88) and might also make you lose some of your good proteins.

The management of ascites and edema is a very difficult task; it requires good judgment and patience, as this will not resolve in one shot but rather needs close monitoring and follow-up.

For my father, a low dosage of spironolactone (Aldactone®) helped to keep his ascites and edema in check most of the time. During the advanced phase of his cancer, we found that support socks helped to reduce the swelling in his lower legs and feet. They are available in different ranges of compression (we used moderate) at most drug stores. We would help him put them on, rolling them up just past his knees. His only complaint was that they were uncomfortably hot sometimes, especially at night. Massaging the feet and ankles is another good way to help maintain flexibility.

88. What is meant when my platelets are low?

Platelets are small cell parts that help the blood to form a clot. Portal hypertension (see Question 87) might also cause blood to back up into the **spleen**, which then starts enlarging to accommodate for the increased

Spleen

an organ located in the upper left part of the abdomen that filters toxic foreign substances from the blood. In case of liver failure, the spleen may enlarge.

blood flow. The spleen typically entraps platelets, and with a larger spleen, more platelets will lodge there. This will lead to a reduced amount of platelets in the blood. In general, not much can be done to improve your platelet count; however, stable and well-controlled cirrhosis and portal hypertension may improve the platelet count somewhat. Alcohol should be completely avoided to prevent the cirrhosis from worsening and further reducing the platelet count.

The low platelet count might limit the kind of diagnostic procedures or therapies that you might be offered because of the increased risk of bleeding. Your doctor might not feel that it is safe to have a biopsy to diagnose your cancer. This is acceptable because with low platelets you might not be eligible to receive an embolization or chemotherapy (e.g., because of the risk of bleeding). Remember that chemotherapy reduces your platelets count (see Question 67). In that instance, caring for your cirrhosis would be of utmost importance.

89. I am vomiting or passing blood or coffee ground material in my stool.

The high pressure buildup caused by portal hypertension might lead to the development of collateral blood vessels called varices in many body organs, such as the esophagus and stomach. These collaterals, however, are at a risk of bleeding as the high pressure is also transmitted through them. The esophageal and stomach varices might open up and bleed, causing you to vomit blood or coffee ground material. You might or might not have bloody or dark stools as well. This is an emergency that requires immediate medical attention. If you witness any of these symptoms, please call your doctor or any emergency medical service immediately.

You might feel a rapid heart beat because your heart is trying to compensate for the lost blood, and you might faint. The bleeding might not stop and might require immediate medical intervention.

90. How can I stop the bleeding?

If you happen to have a variceal bleed, time is of the essence. In the emergency room, you will be transfused with blood and plasma to replace the blood that you lost and to help your blood to clot. Depending on the severity of the episode, your gastroenterologist or hepatologist might elect to perform an endoscopy to locate the bleeding varices and place a rubber band on them in an attempt to prevent recurrence of the bleeding. Other interventions might also be needed. In all instances, you might already have been or you will be prescribed different medications to help reduce your risk of bleeding (blood pressure medications from the beta-blockers family) or to stop the bleeding when it happens (octreolide).

91. I think I am yellow or that my eyes are yellow. What does that mean?

If a mechanical blockage of your bile duct is not present, then jaundice (see Questions 22 and 83) is usually a sign of advanced liver failure or cirrhosis. Liver destruction leads to further accumulation of bile that will show as increased bilirubin and jaundice. As cirrhosis advances, the bilirubin or jaundice worsen (see Question 28). Not much can be done to reverse this jaundice, except possibly liver transplantation (see Question 47). However, your doctor might prescribe antihistamines such as Atarax or Benadryl to ease any itching that you might have. These medications might make you sleepy though. This sleepiness could become important and should be carefully assessed as not to confuse it with any symptoms that are directly related to cirrhosis (see Question 92). Considerable research exists regarding the use of acupuncture to alleviate some of the itching; however, this is still in the research phase. You are encouraged though to discuss it with your doctor.

92. My family or people surrounding me are stating that I am confused sometimes.

The cirrhotic liver might not be able to process many toxic substances, which will accumulate in the blood and may circulate through the brain and alter your mental status. You might be confused or sleepy at times. You might have personality changes. In advanced cases, patients may fall into a **coma**. These symptoms are collectively called encephalopathy. They might happen gradually and over a long period of time or more acutely depending on the evolvement of the liver disease. You and your family should keep your doctor updated regarding any signs or symptoms that relate to disturbed level of awareness, episodes of forgetfulness, confusion, personality changes, seizures, or any other concern you might have because some treatments might help this condition (see Question 93).

Coma

loss of consciousness that may occur when the liver is no longer working well.

93. How can I think more clearly?

To improve the encephalopathy, therapy is aimed to reduce the amount of toxins you might have in your body. **Ammonia** is among the most notorious substances that lead to this condition, but not necessarily the only one. You may be prescribed Lactulose® (or Duphalac®), a laxative that will reduce the amount of protein and nitrogen-based substances absorbed

Ammonia

a body of excreted substances that normally is broken down by the liver.

through your intestines. The amount of lactulose that you need can be gauged by the number of stools that you have per day. You should aim at two to four soft bowel movements per day. In addition, you might be asked to restrict the amount of protein you take for the same reason. This can pose a delicate issue when it comes to balancing your need for nutrition. Your doctor will help you balance the two by prescribing a pre-set amount of protein that you can take per day. Your doctor can follow your improvement not only clinically as your symptoms improve, but also by measuring your blood ammonia level.

PART NINE

Social and End-of-Life Issues

Can my liver cancer be transmitted to my family?

Can I work while getting treated?

What if my doctors suggest stopping my current therapy? What is the best supportive care?

More ...

94. Can my liver cancer be transmitted to my family?

Although the hepatitis virus can be transmitted by patients with active disease, hepatocellular cancer is not contagious. Your family members should be reassured that they will not develop cancer by being around you. If you have a genetic disease that caused your cancer (see Table 3, Question 12), then your children should be screened for the disease. Your doctor should discuss this with you.

95. Can I work while getting treated?

Most patients with primary liver cancer can return to work after surgery, liver transplant, or a local therapy such as embolization. Also, many patients who are receiving chemotherapy can continue going to work. If your body allows and you are not tired, go to work to keep a sense of normalcy in your life. You may be able to work only part time, as you may need a few days after treatment to rest and recover. In all instances, make sure to discuss your interests and concerns with your doctor. If you are working, you are most likely entitled to sick days or even an unpaid leave. You can check the United States Department of Labor Medical Leave Act of 1993 at *http://www.dol.gov/esa/regs/compliance/whd/whdfs28.htm*. You may also need to review your disability benefits. The benefits department at your job should be able to discuss all of the benefits to which you are entitled.

You may be concerned to tell your supervisor or co-workers about your diagnosis of cancer. It is definitely a personal preference regarding how much information you want to share. However, more importantly, you should not fear being treated differently or being discriminated against. The Americans with Disabilities Act clearly states your rights and protects you against discrimination at work. It also requires that employers make reasonable adjustments as long as you can perform the essential functions of your job. You may need to discuss your work schedule, limitations, and other aspects of your job with the human resources department. In case of a conflict, you may need to contact your lawyer or the United States Department of Justice at 800-514-0301 or at *http://www.usdoj.gov/crt/ada/adahom1.htm.*

Remember that your supervisor and co-workers may feel uncomfortable knowing about your diagnosis, either because of previous family experience or because of fear of a disease that they do not know much about. For those who are apt, try to educate them, and for those who decide to alienate you, remain kind and courteous. With time, as they see you functioning like any other person, their fears and anxieties may dissipate and the relationship may normalize.

96. What if my doctors suggest stopping my current therapy? What is the best supportive care?

If the cancer becomes too advanced and resistant to therapy or if your body becomes too weak to tolerate any treatment, your doctor may elect to stop all active therapies. You may be angry or upset or feel helpless about that. However, your doctor is definitely not giving up on you but rather trying to protect you from harm that might affect you badly. Your doctor will then concentrate on alleviating any symptoms that you have. This is called best supportive care. It is an active approach. You will still see your doctor regularly. You will be discussing pain control, nutrition, abdominal distention or leg swelling if any, jaundice, and other symptoms or concerns that you might have. Controlling those symptoms will allow you to maintain some functional level at this stage of your disease. You should use this time to visit your family and friends, visit places you like, enjoy your hobbies, and attend religious services. Keeping a positive and hopeful attitude is the key to succeed through this period of time.

97. What is hospice?

If your medical condition worsens, you may become debilitated and need a lot of help and support. This can be provided through **hospice** care. Hospice is a global care approach that addresses medical, physical, emotional, social, and spiritual needs for patients with advanced-stage disease. This care can be provided at home, especially if your family is around and is able and ready to provide the physical care. You will be visited by a hospice registered nurse and possibly a hospice care physician on a regular basis and as frequently as is necessary. The regular assessments will ensure that you remain comfortable and that all of your needs are addressed. The hospice care team will consult regularly with your doctor. If necessary, you may also be provided with a home health aide care to assist you with your physical needs such as bathing. Although the hospice caring team will be present at your home for only a few hours a day, it will be available 24 hours a day, 7 days a week if need be.

You may also have hospice care provided at a hospice facility as an in-patient because of personal wishes,

Hospice

a facility or program that provides medical, emotional, and spiritual support for terminally ill patients at an inpatient facility or at the patient's home.

family members who need to go to work, or you require strenuous care that your family members cannot provide. At this time of illness, you can still have quality time with your family and loved ones at an in-patient hospice with extended visiting hours. Meanwhile, the staff will provide all of the care that you need.

You are entitled to hospice care after you and your doctor decide not to pursue any further active care like chemotherapy. If your illness appears life threatening at this time, your doctor may also recommend hospice. A hospice program may include palliative care. Additional information is available at *www.hospiceinfo.org* and *www.hospicenet.org*. Some hospice facilities provide palliative care or specific spiritual care. You can discuss with your doctor what options are available or visit the website of the National Hospice and Palliative Care Organization at *www.nhpco.org*.

In addition to giving top-notch care for my father, the hospice provided much needed relief for us, as family. They took care of all of the little things, such as checking up on him during the night, changing his position in bed, and making sure that he took his pain medication. They allowed my mother to rest and recuperate.

At the time, I hated the idea of the hospice because it forced me to come to grips that the care was palliative only and that my father's condition was terminal. However, I could not hate the hospice itself. The nurses were always friendly and attentive, and the condition of the facility was much nicer than the hospital. The hospice that we found was about 10 miles from my sister's home. After 3 days there, my father expressed his wishes to be in a more familiar environment; thus, the hospice helped us transport him to

*my sister's house, where we could be with him during his
final days.*

98. What are advanced directives?

Considering the advanced nature of your cancer, you
may want to direct your caring team in advance about
your wishes. **Advanced directives** are legal documents
that are made to protect your wishes and to make sure
that those are granted. The two basic forms of
advanced directives are a living will and a **healthcare
proxy** (see Question 99).

In a living will, you may state specific instructions that
relate to your medical care in case you are unable to
communicate them. It should state clearly your wishes
in case your heart stops beating or you stop breathing.
Your doctor may offer a short version of a living will
that addresses those two issues. In case of advanced
cancer, your medical condition may worsen enough
that your heart and lungs stop working and die. You
may ask for **cardiopulmonary resuscitation** and have
compressions on your chest, electric shock applied to
your heart, medications infused to speed your heart, a
plastic tube inserted down your throat, and connection
made to a breathing machine. In the case of advanced
cancer, these heroic interventions are more likely to
fail. If anything, they may be tormenting, painful, and
nondignifying to you and your family. In those
instances, your doctor may recommend that you have a
Do-Not-Resuscitate (DNR), Do-Not-Intubate (DNI)
order. Of course, you have the full right to refuse and
still ask for those interventions. Have an open and
frank discussion with your doctor about DNR/DNI
orders to make sure that you understand them fully.

**Advanced
directives**

patient's wishes that
he or she expresses in
advance in regard to
terminal illness.

Healthcare proxy

person assigned by or
designated for a
patient to help make
medical decisions in
the case the patient's
condition does not
allow him or her to
do so.

**Cardiopulmonary
resuscitation**

an emergency proce-
dure in which cardiac
massage, artificial
respiration, and
drugs are used to
regain and maintain
heart and lung func-
tion.

Discuss those wishes in advance and do not leave them till the last minute. When you are comfortable and do not feel pushed, you are more likely to make a rational decision. Remember that a DNR/DNI order does not limit your access to medical care in any way. You may still be receiving chemotherapy but already stated your wishes about end-of-life issues.

Your will might also include wishes that relate to drawing blood, giving blood, feeding, **dialysis**, etc. Make sure that all of this is discussed fully with your doctor. Generally, your doctor will not recommend any invasive measures, except if it truly will improve your survival. Otherwise, he or she will guide you to make a decision that would improve your comfort. Remember that sometimes in medicine doing less is doing more.

Dialysis
clearing blood of toxins by passing it through machines, in case of kidney failure.

The other part of the advanced directive is to assign a healthcare proxy. You may need to do that, and it is highly recommended either because some states do not recognize living wills or because some decisions not previously discussed with you need to be made while you are asleep, unconscious, or simply unable to make them. In those instances, your healthcare proxy (also called a health surrogate, a medical proxy, or a medical power of attorney) will act on your behalf and make those decisions.

A healthcare proxy should be someone that you trust and someone you know and believe will make decisions based on your wishes stated and not stated. This can be a family member or a friend. Make sure to inform your healthcare proxy of interest about your wish to assign them. Make sure that he or she is comfortable with that decision, and if so, make sure to lead a candid and honest discussion about your wishes. It is also important that you inform your friends and family about who is your healthcare proxy in order to avoid any unnecessary conflict that may arise at some tense moments. You can discuss healthcare proxy issues with your caring team, the social worker, patient representative, or your lawyer.

99. What should I do to prepare to die? Where is hope?

Although death is a fearful reality, preparing for it might help to make it a smooth transition. You should never believe that thinking of death means giving up. It is rather an opportunity that helps you shape how your life will end. The earlier that you prepare the better, as you do not want to feel pressured or disappointed if things do not go the way you wish.

Clear your financial issues. Work with your attorney, accountant, and your family. You may need to write a will, especially if you have family that is financially dependent on you. Sort out your financial plan and keep your attorney name and contacts available. Also, keep all legal, financial, or health documents organized for easier access.

See your loved ones, family, friends, and colleagues. Talk to people who live far away. If you are troubled by any unresolved issues with somebody, work on sorting them out. Indicate to whom you want to give any valuable items you have. Collectibles and photographs are memories that will celebrate your life and may be passed from one generation to another. Depending on your beliefs, you may wish to prepare some aspects of your funeral. This is a celebration of your life and an important closure for everybody.

The biggest fear that remains is leaving your loved ones behind, especially children. See them as often as you can. Prepare an album of photos about moments of your life that you would like to share with them. Leave for them any scrapbooks or diaries.

As you can imagine, you might still be busy even close to your death. Remember and recite to yourself your dearest moments. You will notice that you are abundant with life.

One of my closest friends, Francis, lost his father to liver cancer shortly before I did. He told me the best advice ever. Tell your father you love him for everything he has done. Do it early and often. I am glad I listened to him. In the few days before he passed away, my father had trouble speaking due to encephalopathy, and thus, I could only be there to comfort him. It is very important to communicate as much as possible before the illness becomes too advanced.

100. Where can I find more information?

Throughout the book, we mention several other resources that might help you to get more information or answers to your questions. In the computer age, the Internet is a great resource to many aspects of your liver cancer. Generally, the information is periodically updated.

You have to exert caution, however, as some Internet sites may have information that is not verified. Always check with your healthcare team if you are in doubt. Chat rooms could be another resource that helps you share your experience and exchange information. Remember, however, that no two patients are alike, and thus, treat this information critically before acting on it. A comprehensive cancer center can have many resources available to you as well. Always make sure to ask because you will be amazed how much care and support are available.

Glossary

α-Fetoprotein: a blood marker that may be elevated in primary liver cancer

Abdominal distention: bulging of the belly.

Ablation: the destruction of a tumor without actually removing it. Examples include heating (radiofrequency ablation), freezing (cryotherapy), injecting a toxic substance such as ethanol or chemotherapy, or decreasing its blood supply, as in hepatic artery embolization.

Abscess: a collection of pus

Acupuncture: a Chinese medical procedure in which fine needles are placed through the skin to relieve pain or for other treatment reasons

Acute viral hepatitis: an active infection caused by a hepatitis virus

Adefovir: an antiviral drug that is used for patients with chronic hepatitis B

Adjuvant therapy: a form of therapy that will help prevent the recurrence of cancer after a potentially curative treatment such as surgery

Advanced directives: patient's wishes that he or she expresses in advance in regard to terminal illness

Aflatoxins: a group of molds that contaminate stored food supplies and may lead to cirrhosis and ultimately liver cancer

Alcohol injection: inserting alcohol through a needle into a tumor. This technique is widely used to treat small hepatomas. Alcohol is directly toxic to the tumor.

Alcoholic liver disease: liver cirrhosis caused by excessive alcohol ingestion

Alternative medicine: medical practices (e.g., herbal medicine) that do not follow Western medicine guidelines and may lack scientific proof for their effectiveness

Ammonia: a body of excreted substances that normally is broken down by the liver

Anesthesia: medication that puts someone to sleep and/or reduces pain

Anesthesiologist: a doctor who specializes in the delivery of anesthesia

Antibiotics: medications used to fight infections

Aorta: the largest artery in the body. It originates from the heart, and its branches supply the entire body with blood containing oxygen.

Arteriography: a radiologic test that demonstrates the artery branches of a person. The technique is performed by an interventional radiologist. Typically, a small tube is inserted into the patient's leg during the procedure. A contrast agent is injected, and x-rays are then taken to reveal the arteries. Arteriography is used to identify the artery branches that supply a tumor during hepatic artery embolization.

Ascites: an abnormal accumulation of fluid in the abdomen

Bile: a collection of salts and proteins that is made by the liver and carried by the bile duct to the gallbladder and the intestine. Bile is green and gives feces their brown color.

Bilirubin: a component of bile that comes from the breakdown of red blood cells

Biopsy: the physical sampling of a piece of tissue. In patients with a suspected tumor, a biopsy is used to determine whether the patient has a cancer and what type of tumor it is.

A biopsy is generally performed by passing a needle through the skin into a tumor.

Body surface area: a measurement used to dose chemotherapy based on a patient's height and weight

Bone marrow: substance that fills the bone inner cavities and is the source of red blood cells, white blood cells, and platelets

Brachytherapy: radiation therapy that is applied within the body cavity

Cancer: the uncontrolled replication of cells that leads to abnormal growth that may invade local organs or tissues or may travel to other places in the body

Cardiopulmonary resuscitation: an emergency procedure in which cardiac massage, artificial respiration, and drugs are used to regain and maintain heart and lung function

Cells: the smallest structural unit of a living organism that is capable of functioning independently

Ceruloplasmin: a protein that binds to copper

Chemotherapy: chemical agents that are used to treat cancer

Child Pugh score: a score used to assess the level of cirrhosis

Cholangiocarcinoma: cancer of the bile ducts

Chronic viral hepatitis: continuous state of infection during which the liver continues to be inflamed and may ultimately cause cirrhosis and cancer.

Cirrhosis: condition in which normal liver tissue is replaced with scarred tissue. It is often associated with varied levels of loss of liver functions.

Clinical trial: a research study that answers many of the questions regarding newly discovered therapies

Coma: loss of consciousness that may occur when the liver is no longer working well

Complementary medicine (same as alternative medicine): medical practices (e.g., herbal medicine) that do not follow Western medicine guidelines and that may lack a scientific proof for their effectiveness

Computed tomography (CT scan): a form of x-ray images in which acquired images are constructed by computer to form cross-sectional images of the body

Creatinine: a substance usually excreted from the body through urine. It is used to help assess kidney function

Cryotherapy: a form of therapy that uses cold temperature to kill cancer cells

Cytotoxic drugs: chemical substances that are used as chemotherapy to kill cancer cells

Depression: a sad state of mind characterized by feeling tired, with an inability to concentrate, an inability to sleep, a decreased appetite, guilt, and thoughts of death. Although it may be a psychiatric illness, it also may occur to patients facing a serious illness, such as primary liver cancer or other forms of cancer.

Diabetes: a disease condition in which the body is unable to control sugar levels. In some instances, diabetes may lead to multiple complications and other diseases, and possibly primary liver cancer.

Dialysis: clearing blood of toxins by passing it through machines, in case of kidney failure

Diuretics (water pills): drugs that increase the discharge of urine

Echocardiogram: a test for the heart in which pictures and functional values of the heart are obtained using ultrasound

Edema: an abnormal accumulation of fluid in the extremities

Electrocardiogram: an electrical tracing of the heart

Encephalopathy: an altered sense of consciousness. It may occur when the liver is not working well. The patient may seemed confused or have inappropriate social behavior. It may vary in severity from day to day.

Endoscopy: a procedure performed by a gastroenterologist. A tube is placed into your mouth while you are lightly sedated. The doctor can then look at the inside of the stomach and the first part of the intestine to search for dilated blood vessels (varices), ulcers, or gastritis.

External beam radiation: radiation therapy that is aimed at a specific site in the body and delivered from outside of the body through the skin

Fatigue: physical tiredness

Fatty liver: condition in which fat accumulates in the liver because of a liver illness caused by one of several diseases (e.g., viral hepatitis)

Fibrolamellar hepatocellular carcinoma: a variant of hepatoma that occurs typically in young adults. It generally has a more favorable outcome and is not associated with underlying liver disease.

Foley catheter: a tube that is placed into the bladder to monitor precisely the urine output of a patient.

Fungus: a type of organism than can cause an infection

Gallbladder: a storage tank for bile. It is attached to the liver. It squeezes the bile into your intestine when you eat a fatty meal.

Gastritis: inflammation of the inside lining of the stomach

Gastroenterologist: a person who specializes in the treatment of diseases that affect the gastrointestinal system, including the liver, stomach, and pancreas

Healthcare proxy: person assigned by or designated for a patient to help make medical decisions in the case the patient's condition does not allow him or her to do so

Hematoma: a collection of blood

Hemochromatosis: a hereditary disease that leads to excessive accumulation of iron in the body and may cause liver disease and ultimately primary liver cancer

Hepatic artery: the blood vessel that carries oxygenated blood to the liver

Hepatic artery embolization: the injection of microscopic particles (either attached to a chemotherapy drug or not) into the branches of the hepatic artery in order to ablate or destroy a liver tumor. The treatment works by blocking the blood supply to the tumor and, when chemotherapy is used, by delivering chemotherapy to the tumor.

Hepatitis: inflammation of the liver. It may be caused by a variety of agents, including viruses, excessive alcohol use, metabolic diseases, and environmental toxins

Hepatobiliary surgeon: a doctor who specializes in the surgical and ablative treatments of liver, gallbladder, bile duct, and pancreas tumors

Hepatoblastoma: a rare type of primary liver cancer that occurs in children

Hepatocellular cancer: a type of primary liver cancer that originates in hepatocytes; a type of liver cell.

Hepatocellular carcinoma: cancer of the liver cells, a type of primary liver cancer

Hepatocytes: liver cells

Hepatologist: a liver disease specialist

Hepatoma: short name for hepatocellular cancer

Homeopathy: treating disease with small amounts of treatments that in large amounts in healthy people may produce symptoms of the same disease. This is a medical practice that is based on resemblance between the drug and the disease.

Hospice: a facility or program that provides medical, emotional, and spiritual support for terminally ill patients at an inpatient facility or at the patient's home

Human immunodeficiency virus (HIV): a virus that destroys helper cells of the immune system that usually fight infections and may lead to AIDS

Immune system: an intricate body system that protects people against foreign organisms or toxins that may cause disease

Inferior vena cava: a large vein that is supplied by multiple veins from the lower parts of the body and helps bring the blood back to the heart

Institutional review board: a collective board that oversees all clinical trials. The board generally includes doctors, researchers, lawyers, administrators, pharmacists, and patients' advocates.

Integrative medicine: a discipline that is used to treat patients using modern science and alternative medicine

Interferon-α: a protein that is produced by specific cells in response to infection or cancer in an aim to protect the body. It is used to treat hepatitis.

Interventional radiologist: a doctor who specializes in performing procedures under radiologic (ultrasound, x-ray, or CT scan) guidance such as

tumor biopsies, hepatic artery embolization, or a metaport

Intestine: the part of the gastrointestinal tract between the stomach and rectum. The intestine helps digest food and regulate water, certain vitamins, and salts of the body.

Jaundice: yellowish discoloration of the skin and eyes caused by accumulation of bilirubin

Kidneys: two organs located in the abdomen that are responsible for water and electrolytes balance, and that help excrete body metabolites through urine

Lamivudine: an antivirus drug that is commonly used against HIV and also against hepatitis C

Laparoscopy: a procedure that is done under general anesthesia and performed by a surgeon in which the inside of the abdomen can be examined through a few small incisions

Liver: an organ located in the upper right-hand side of the abdomen; responsible for making proteins and removing toxins and wastes from the body

Liver capsule: the outside lining of the liver. It is the only part of the liver that can trigger a sensation of pain.

Liver resection: the surgical removal of all or a portion of the liver

Local anesthetic: numbing medication that is injected directly at the site where a procedure is to be performed

Lymph nodes: small bodies along the lymphatic system that supply a special kind of fighter white blood cells called lymphocytes to the bloodstream. They are also responsible for removing bacteria and foreign particles from the lymph. Lymph nodes may be invaded by cancer and may also help transmitting cancer to other sites o f the body. Lymph nodes are also known as lymph glands.

Magnetic resonance imaging (MRI): a form of radiologic imaging that uses magnetic fields to produce electronic images of the inner parts of the human body

Mediport: a half-dollar sized, round well that is connected to a tube that is used for the delivery of medication within a vein. The entire apparatus sits underneath the skin and is inserted during a small procedure.

MELD (model for end-stage liver disease): a mathematical equation that is used to prioritize patients for liver transplantation based on their laboratory values

Metabolic diseases: diseases in which the metabolism of a certain product may be impaired. They are usually genetically inherited.

Metastasis: the spread of cancer beyond its primary location

Multiple gated acquisition scan (MUGA): a noninvasive test that produces a moving image of the heart and assesses function level

Naturopathy: the science that uses herbs and herb products as a form of therapy against disease

Nausea: the feeling of sickness in the stomach with an urge to vomit

Neoadjuvant therapy: therapy that is given before surgical removal of a cancer, aiming at reducing its size and rendering it more resectable

Nerve: a type of tissue in the body that can transmit sensations such as pain, pressure, or temperature

Nonalcoholic fatty liver disease: disease that leads to the development of fatty liver by injuries other than excessive alcohol use

Nonsteroidal anti-inflammatory drugs: a form of medication that controls pain and inflammation that is not part of the steroid family

Oncologists: medical doctor specialists who treat cancer

Partial hepatectomy: the surgical removal of part of the liver

Pathologist: a doctor who specializes in the diagnosis of diseases of the body by evaluating biopsies from the disease site, like cancer

Pathology laboratory: the section of the hospital in which a pathologist works and where tissue specimens are analyzed

Pathology report: a typed report issued by a pathologist that describes the results of the analysis of a biopsy or surgical specimen

Pathology slides: 3 × 1 inch glass slides on which tissue from a biopsy or a surgical specimen is placed

Peripheral edema: excessive accumulation of fluids in the legs that leads to swelling

Platelets: pieces of cells that float in the blood and promote clotting where necessary

Pneumonia: a lung infection

Portal hypertension: increased pressure within the veins of the liver, which can lead to poor liver function, increased size of the spleen, and consequently, a low platelet count, or varices (dilated veins of the stomach or esophagus)

Portal vein: a blood vessel that carries blood from the intestines to within the liver

Primary liver cancer: cancer that originates within the liver

Proteins: essential body substances that include enzymes, hormones, antibodies, and other substances that are critical for the functioning of the human body

Prothrombin: a protein produced by the liver that helps blood to clot

Protocol: a detailed description of all of the rules and conditions that govern a clinical trial. A protocol is the ultimate reference for a clinical trial.

Pump: a pump system used to deliver chemotherapy at a fixed rate and for a specific period of time

Radiation: a ray of powerful energy that is emitted from a radioactive material

Radiation hepatitis: inflammatory damage to the liver that may be caused by radiation therapy

Radiation therapy: treatment against cancer that uses radiation as a form of energy to kill cancer cells

Radioactive lipiodol embolization: a procedure in which the blood vessels of the liver tumor are clogged by injecting them with the inert substance lipiodol that is tagged to radioactive material as an additional form of therapy

Radiofrequency ablation: a form of tumor ablation that relies on heating to destroy tumor cells. It may be performed by inserting a metal probe through the skin into a liver tumor. Alternatively, it may be performed at the time of laparoscopy or laparotomy (open surgical exploration).

Radiologists: doctors who specialize in interpreting x-rays, CTs, MRIs, and other radiologic tests

Red blood cells: cells that carry oxygen and carbon dioxide. They are red because of their high load of iron, which is essential to their function.

Rejection: the process by which the body refuses a donated transplanted liver and regards it as foreign

Ribavirin: an antiviral drug used against hepatitis C

Screening: studies and evaluations that attempt to identify a predisease state or an early form of disease, aiming at controlling it before it becomes advanced

Secondary liver cancer: cancers that started in other organs of the body and have traveled to the liver

Somatostatin analogues: variants of a hormonal protein that may be used to prevent the recurrence of primary liver cancer

Spleen: an organ located in the upper left part of the abdomen that filters toxic foreign substances from the blood. In case of liver failure, the spleen may enlarge.

Staging system: a set of definitions that allows physicians to define the extent of a certain cancer and recommend therapy accordingly

Thrombosis: the formation of clots

Tolerance: the body's need for an increased dose of a certain medication to obtain the same effect

Transplantation: the removal of a patient's entire liver and replacement with part or all of the liver from another person. The other person may be alive (live donor) or just deceased (cadaveric donor).

Triphasic CT: a CT scan that evaluates the liver at three phases of the blood flow through it

Tumor: a cancerous growth

Ulcer: a lesion of the stomach that results from inflammation and may bleed

Ultrasound: the use of ultrasonic waves to view images of an internal body structure

Varix: an abnormally swollen vein that is prone to bleed

Variceal bleed: an actively bleeding varix, which is a dilated vein

Viral hepatitis: inflammatory condition of the liver caused by an infection with a hepatitis virus

White blood cells: cells that help fight infection

Wilson's disease: an inherited disease of impaired copper metabolism

Yttrium-90 microspheres: small beads tagged with radioactive Yttrium that are delivered into the liver and lodge inside the small arteries to deliver their anticancer therapeutic effect

Index

Staging system, 27, 30
Supportive care, 105–106
Surgery. *See* Liver resection

T

Targeted therapies, 75
Therasopheres, 79–80
Thrombosis, 57
Tolerance, 92
Transplantation, 9. *See also* Liver transplantation
Treatment. *See* Liver cancer treatment
Triphasic CT, 70
Tumors. *See also* Liver resection
  ablation of, 38, 59
  explanation of, 2
  growth patterns of, 24–25
  method for staging, 27
  removal of, 40–41
  return of, 51
  screening for, 18, 19
Tylenol®, *See* Acetaminophen

U

Ulcers, 47
Ultrasound
  to evaluate chemotherapy treatment, 70
  to evaluate for liver transplantation, 55

explanation of, 19, 20
United Network for Organ Sharing (UNOS), 53, 54

V

Variceal bleeds, 22, 98–99
Varices, 47
Veterans Affairs Department, 35
Viral hepatitis. *See also* Hepatitis
  acute, 9–10
  chronic, 8, 10, 12–13, 16
  explanation of, 8
  following liver transplantation, 52
  transmission of, 104
Vitamin A, 50

W

White blood cells, 72, 73
Wilson's disease, 14

Y

Yttrium-90 microspheres, 79–80